the**facts**

prostate cancer

Also available in the**facts** series

the**facts**

prostate
cancer

SECOND EDITION

MALCOLM MASON

Cancer Research Wales Professor of
Clinical Oncology
Cardiff University

LESLIE MOFFAT

Consultant Urological Surgeon and Honorary
Senior Lecturer
University of Aberdeen

9/10

OXFORD
UNIVERSITY PRESS

OXFORD
UNIVERSITY PRESS

Great Clarendon Street, Oxford OX2 6DP

Oxford University Press is a department of the University of Oxford.
It furthers the University's objective of excellence in research, scholarship,
and education by publishing worldwide in

Oxford New York

Auckland Cape Town Dar es Salaam Hong Kong Karachi
Kuala Lumpur Madrid Melbourne Mexico City Nairobi
New Delhi Shanghai Taipei Toronto

With offices in

Argentina Austria Brazil Chile Czech Republic France Greece
Guatemala Hungary Italy Japan Poland Portugal Singapore
South Korea Switzerland Thailand Turkey Ukraine Vietnam

Oxford is a registered trade mark of Oxford University Press
in the UK and in certain other countries

Published in the United States
by Oxford University Press Inc., New York

British Library Cataloguing in Publication Data

Data available

Library of Congress Cataloging in Publication Data

Typeset in Plantin
by Glyph International, Bangalore, India
Printed in Great Britain by Ashford Colour Press Ltd., Gosport, Hampshire

ISBN 978–0–19–957393–6

10 9 8 7 6 5 4 3 2 1

Whilst every effort has been made to ensure that the contents of this book are as complete,
accurate and up-to-date as possible at the date of writing, Oxford University Press is not
able to give any guarantee or assurance that such is the case. Readers are urged to take
appropriately qualified medical advice in all cases. The information in this book is intended
to be useful to the general reader, but should not be used as a means of self-diagnosis or for
the prescription of medication.

Foreword

As a lay member of a cancer research group, I was very impressed by the standard of this publication. It provides an excellent bridge between the information leaflets given at the time of diagnosis, and the technical descriptions of prostate cancer and its treatments that are found in medical and scientific journals and textbooks. The elements of prostate cancer and its biology, diagnosis, and treatment are clearly laid out and expertly described. Other chapters describing management options, research trials and screening evaluation are clear and concise, but of sufficient detail to inform the enquiring reader. The book is easily navigated, and logically constructed. I can thoroughly recommend it to anyone seeking clear answers to many of the pertinent questions which are raised by prostate cancer patients and their families, and also by middle aged men of a certain disposition, of which I number one.

David Ardron
Chair
National Cancer Research Institute Consumer Liaison Group
North Trent Cancer Research Network Consumer Research Panel
May 2010

Preface to the First Edition

Prostate cancer has become one of the commonest male cancers in the Western world. There is a plethora of information about the disease, especially on the Internet. In some instances, there is a 'spin' or 'hype' imparted to the information that is unhelpful or even may be unethical. In this book, we have, as two practising doctors, one an oncologist and the other a surgeon, tried to give the information about this complex disease as it really is, without bias.

This is a book for those patients and their carers who wish to go beyond the patient leaflets that are now, fortunately, readily available. Medical information can be impenetrable at worst or inaccessible at best. More detailed explanations of certain aspects are given here, in the hope that the interested layperson can begin to penetrate medical thinking, be guided through a morass of data, and to allow them to arrive at an informed position. Some degree of repetition is inevitable in this book—patients with prostate cancer vary so much that not all chapters will be relevant to all patients, and those dipping into different, selected chapters will hopefully find the information that they need without too much cross-referencing.

We hope that, through this book, we can in some small way help society as a whole to take stock of the dilemma that is prostate cancer.

Malcolm Mason
Leslie Moffat
2003

Preface to the Second Edition

In the years since the first edition was published there have been a number of extremely important advances. The first randomized trials of screening have been published; an important randomized trial has compared surgery and watchful waiting for the first time. In advanced disease, a number of new treatment options have become available, notably chemotherapy, and many more are waiting in the wings.

Despite these advances, many controversies remain, and, unlike some other types of cancer, men with prostate cancer often have several treatment options open to them which can be difficult to choose between.

We believe that men with prostate cancer, and their families, deserve the opportunity to make an informed choice about whether or not to be screened, and, if they are diagnosed with prostate cancer, how they will be treated. It is our intention that this book should arm them with some of the necessary information, and equip them as we ourselves would wish to be equipped in similar circumstances.

Malcolm Mason
Leslie Moffat
November 2009

Contents

1

Introduction

➜ Key points

◆ Many men do not know where the prostate gland is, or what its function is in the body.

◆ Most men have enlargement of the prostate gland from middle age onwards, a condition called 'benign prostatic hyperplasia' or BPH.

◆ BPH can cause problems in urinating; prostate cancer, by contrast, often produces no symptoms when it is relatively small, and confined to the inside of the prostate.

◆ Problems with urination are uncommonly caused by prostate cancer.

'They kept on saying that there was a tumour in the prostate; I didn't fully understand, but finally I plucked up the courage and asked the doctor "Is it cancer?", and he said yes. It was quite a shock, of course, but he was very honest with me, and at least I could start trying to come to terms with it.'

The prostate—what is it, where is it, and how is it assessed?

The prostate is a gland located just below the bladder in men (Figure 1.1). It is not found in women. It should be noted that the word is 'prostate' and

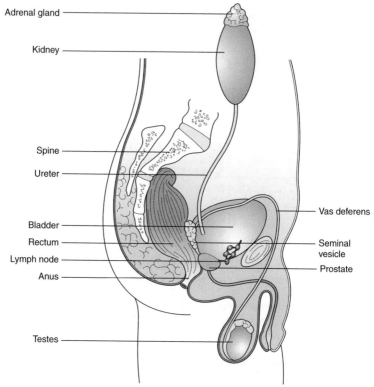

Figure 1.1 Location of the prostate.

not 'prostate'. Its function is imperfectly understood, but seems to be entirely linked to human reproduction. It produces substances that are used to nourish the sperm in semen, and which affect the degree of viscosity of the semen (turning it into a jelly and then later on back into a fluid). It is the best source of hormones called 'prostaglandins', which were first isolated from prostatic tissue. Prostatic secretions may also have an effect on the female reproductive tract.

The seminal vesicles lie alongside the prostate and look like small bunches of grapes. They produce over half the volume of the ejaculate, producing substances such as sugars that nourish the sperm and activate them prior to ejaculation. They drain into the lower area of the prostate. They are usually removed by the operation termed a radical prostatectomy (discussed later in this book), or if necessary treated by radical radiotherapy (also discussed later).

The vas deferens is a tube that joins the testicles to the interior of the prostate. The sperm are released through the ejaculatory duct in the centre of the urethra, which travels through the centre of the prostate. There is a vas on both sides to drain both testicles.

The nerves that control erection of the penis lie at the sides of the prostate. These nerves can be damaged during treatment for prostate cancer, resulting in impotence.

During embryonic development, the prostate wraps itself around the urethra, the tube draining the bladder. Therefore it becomes understandable why, if the prostate gland enlarges, it can cause obstruction to the flow of urine.

Almost all men have a degree of enlargement of the prostate, which is called 'benign prostatic hyperplasia' (BPH). BPH starts in middle age or even earlier. The reasons are still not understood, but the male hormone testosterone is implicated as such enlargement would not occur if a male is castrated before the age of 12. Milder degrees of BPH may produce little or nothing in the way of symptoms, but, if you are affected, BPH can produce a variety of symptoms including hesitancy (having to wait to start urinating), frequency (wanting to urinate more often than usual), or having to get up at night to pass urine.

In a young man of 16, the prostate is slightly bigger than a small walnut. In a man of 80 it can be as large as an orange. Although the prostate is situated deep within the pelvis, it is fortuitous that its back portion can be felt through the rectum (the 'back passage') and this is the basis for the examination whereby a doctor or nurse places his or her gloved finger into your rectum. Two things about the prostate can be assessed by this examination: first, the size of the prostate and, secondly, the consistency of the prostate, which can sometimes indicate cancer of the prostate.

Cancer of the prostate generally feels very hard. Occasionally a small nodule can be felt on the prostate and this can be displayed by taking an image using 'transrectal ultrasound' (TRUS). TRUS also takes advantage of the proximity of the prostate and the rectum. A TRUS probe is inserted into the rectum, taking the place of the doctor's finger. Ultrasonic waves are used to produce a picture on a screen which can indicate the presence of a cancer and/or guide a needle used to take biopsy samples of the prostate. This is discussed in more detail elsewhere, but a hypoechoic area (meaning that the area does not produce an echo with the same intensity as the remainder of the prostate) is often associated with malignancy.

Usually, if a TRUS is done, biopsies will be taken. This is done by inserting a needle through the probe, usually taking eight to ten samples but sometimes more. A biopsy will only be taken after you have received antibiotics, given either by injection or as tablets, and further antibiotics may be given later, after the biopsy. Often, you will receive a local anaesthetic injection through the rectum before the biopsies are actually taken, as in many men this might make the whole procedure less uncomfortable. An expert pathologist can determine from the biopsy sample of the prostate whether or not cancer is present, and if it is, the **grade** of the cancer. This is an important feature which is discussed in Chapter 2.

The body is composed of many billions of cells organized into tissues and organs. Nature has decreed that animals, including humans, develop and maintain their structure by allowing cells the ability to divide and grow, to replace cells that die after injury or after they have reached their allotted life span. It is a miracle that so few of these cells go off the track. Most behave and live ordinary lives, growing, dividing, and then dying when appropriate. Every day, millions of such cell divisions are taking place in the human body. An essential part of this process is the replication of a cell's entire DNA content—the genetic 'blueprint' for human life. This process is rather like copying the contents of a huge computer 'hard disk' but is vastly more complicated and is not error free. It is estimated that, just as computers make mistakes when files are copied, every day in every person several thousand 'mistakes' are made during cell division. The miracle is that, every day, each of these mistakes is detected and dealt with, but just occasionally one slips through the net.

Occasionally, such a mistake, if uncorrected, allows cells to start developing abnormally and finding a way of bypassing normal control mechanisms. This allows the number of cells in a particular area to grow in an uncontrolled way that could lead to cancer. Nearly all cancers start as a series of mistakes, and arise from just one cell. However, most 'mistakes' will have no effect or, at worst, lead to a benign growth that is not a cancer.

Benign (non-cancerous) enlargement of the prostate (also called 'benign prostatic hyperplasia')

Not all 'growths' arise because of mistakes during DNA replication at cell division. Some result from a change in the normal balance of factors, including hormones such as testosterone, that encourage the healthy growth of an organ such as the prostate. This occurs in other hormone-responsive organs, including the breast in women where the hormone is oestrogen.

Benign enlargement of the prostate with age has already been referred to. Under the microscope it can be seen that the vast majority of this enlargement is due to an increase in the number of cells. This is called 'benign prostatic hyperplasia' (BPH). Despite the increase in the number of cells, this condition is entirely benign or non-malignant.

Malignancy or cancer—which is it?

Malignancy and cancer mean the same thing. Very often, the word 'tumour' is used. Strictly speaking, a tumour may be benign or malignant; it is a good word to use once it is clear whether your condition is benign or whether you have prostate cancer. If you are in any doubt, ask the doctor to be quite clear about it—a direct question, such as 'Do I have cancer of the prostate?' may be a good way of ensuring that you understand, and the doctor knows that you understand, exactly what the situation is. In this book, when we refer to a 'tumour', we mean a cancer.

As discussed, in BPH, the number of cells increases. Despite this, there is still a degree of order in the increased number of cells, and although the prostate may continue to grow, its cells show no signs of leaving their companion cells or attempting to go elsewhere by invading any other areas of the body.

In malignancy, two processes occur.

Invasion

The first process is **invasion**. Cells which have become malignant start to invade the area outside their normal territory. They can invade blood vessels, but in the prostate, they also particularly tend to invade along the channels of the nerves in the prostate. Such cells are able to move outside the capsule of the prostate, resulting in local advancement, or 'progession', of the cancer.

Metastasis

The other hallmark of malignancy is the capacity of the cancer cells, which have left their normal position, to set up colonies in more remote parts of the body. This is **metastasis**—the formation of 'secondaries'. These colonies continue to grow in size and number, and begin to damage normal cells in the areas to which they have spread.

In prostate cancer, such spread occurs to lymph nodes and elsewhere, but prostate cancer cells have a peculiarly close relationship with bone cells, which explains why bone metastases are such a common pattern of spread. Bone metastases can be identified by plain X-rays or bone scans.

Geographical aspects of prostate cancer

Prostate cancer is common in all Western countries, particularly in the USA (Table 1.1). It is particularly common in the black population of North America, where the disease tends to present about 10 years earlier than it would in North American whites. The reason for this unfortunate fact is as yet obscure, but is probably related to a genetic component.

Table 1.1 Age-standardized incidence rates per 100,000 for cancer of the prostate

Country	Incidence
USA: black	137.0
USA, Hawaii: white	108.2
USA: white	100.8
Canada	64.7
USA, Hawaii Japanese	64.2
USA, Hawaii, Chinese	62.9
Zimbabwe, Harare: European	55.7
Sweden	55.3
USA, Puerto Rico	54.7
South Australia	53.6
Austria, Tyrol	51.6
France, Calvados	50.5
USA, Hawaii: Filipino	49.5
USA, Hawaii: Hawaiian	42.1
Finland	41.3
The Netherlands	39.6
Germany: Saarland	35.9
Brazil, Goiania	35.2
Uruguay, Montevideo	32.6

Table 1.1 Age-standardized incidence rates per 100,000 for cancer of the prostate (*continued*)

Country	Incidence
UK, Scotland	31.2
Denmark	31.0
Ireland, Southern	30.9
Zimbabwe, Harare: African	29.2
UK, England and Wales	28.0
Italy, Genoa	24.7
Czech Republic	24.1
Israel: all Jews	23.9
Germany: eastern states	23.7
Ecuador, Quito	22.4
Spain, Zaragoza	19.7
Peru, Lima	19.4
Kuwait: non-Kuwaitis	18.3
Philippines, Manila	17.6
Argentina, Concordia	16.2
Poland, Warsaw City	15.7
Serbia, Vojvodina	14.7
Japan, Hiroshima	10.9
Israel: non-Jews	10.4
Singapore: Chinese	9.8
Hong Kong	7.9
India: Bombay	7.9
Kuwait: Kuwaitis	6.5
China, Shanghai	2.3
Viet Nam: Hanoi	1.2
Korea: Kangwa	0.9

The causes of prostate cancer

There are a number of risk factors. Ageing (particularly over 70 years) is thought to be the strongest risk factor, and there is no doubt that as a population becomes more elderly the incidence rates of prostate cancer also increase in that population.

This contributes to an impression that prostate cancer is becoming more common, an impression which may be exaggerated by the ageing population. Age *per se* is not a cause of prostate cancer. It is simply that the longer a man lives, the more chance his prostate's cells have of going awry. There is another reason why prostate cancer appears to be becoming more common; since the prostate-specific antigen (PSA) test was introduced, many more cancers have been diagnosed which otherwise might never have been discovered and, bizarrely (and prostate cancer may be unique in this sense), might never have caused any harm. Whether detecting these extra cancers is a good thing or not is still extremely controversial.

Diet

The more animal fats that are consumed by a nation, the greater the risk of prostate cancer in its men. Vegetarians are said to be at a much lower risk of developing prostate cancer, perhaps by as much as 50 per cent. The body's fat content affects the handling of testosterone and this may be the link between fat and prostate cancer.

Chinese and Japanese men have a much lower rate of prostate cancer than North Americans and Europeans. There is also an interesting observation that the risk of prostate cancer in Japanese men who have moved from Japan to North America increases towards that of the local population.

It is difficult to disentangle the effects of diet from those of genetic make-up. Prostate cancer is more common in countries where the risk of heart disease is higher, but both could be due to a mixture of dietary and genetic effects.

Possible protective factors in diet

Antioxidants Oxygen is ubiquitous in the human body. The laws of chemistry result in a tendency for complex biological molecules to have oxygen added to them—a process called 'oxidation'. Paradoxically, and despite the fact that oxygen is essential to fuel human life, oxidation damages complex biological materials, including DNA, and may be one factor causing cancer. A number of substances found in food can counteract this effect. Therefore they are called 'antioxidants'. Examples of antioxidants are given in Table 1.2.

Table 1.2 Examples of antioxidants

Vitamin E (the most important natural antioxidant, acts with selenium)	Found in margarine
Vitamin A (beta-carotene)	Found in carrots
Vitamin C	Found in fresh fruit and vegetables

Lycopenes, which are found in cooked tomatoes, may have a mild protective effect but this remains to be proved beyond all reasonable doubt.

Various diets have been devised, and the effect of adding compounds such as retinoids, carotenoids, and vitamin C to an adequate diet continues to be discussed.

Selenium, which is an essential trace element found in plants, enters the food chain by plant ingestion and is essentially dependent on soil concentration. Selenium may protect against the action of certain carcinogens but, very disappointingly, a clinical trial investigating the addition of selenium to the diet showed no evidence that it prevents prostate cancer.

Soya products are said to inhibit prostate cancer. The compounds thought to be responsible are called 'isoflavonoids'.

Industrial exposure

Exposure to cadmium, which can occur in men working in copper smelting, seems to increase the risk of prostate cancer. Some authors have claimed that exposure to ultraviolet light increases the risk of prostate cancer, but this is far from proven. In general, though, it is unlikely that industrial or occupational exposure is responsible for the vast majority of prostate cancers.

Sexual behaviour

There have been a number of studies to investigate whether the younger that a man becomes sexually active, the more he will increase his risk of prostate cancer. The hypothesis is that such men will have had multiple partners and may have been exposed to more viruses than others. However, there is no firm evidence linking sexually acquired viruses with prostate cancer, and on current evidence there is nothing that one can do to modify sexual lifestyle that will reduce the risk of prostate cancer.

Other factors

In recent years, some clinical trials have looked at drugs called '5-alpha reductase inhibitors', which affect the processing of testosterone in the prostate. There are suggestions that the use of these drugs might prevent the formation of some prostate cancers, but they are still under investigation, and it will be important to determine whether or not they might actually reduce the death rate from prostate cancer in the population.

2

How do doctors measure the severity and extent of a prostate cancer?

Key points

- The extent of a prostate cancer is determined by a combination of physical examination, scanning with ultrasound, CT or MRI, and a bone scan.

- The classification used to describe tumour extent is called the TNM system, and all patients should have a TNM category assigned to their prostate cancer.

- The PSA level also reflects the severity of a prostate cancer, and is closely related to its extent.

- Prostate cancer severity is also graded using the Gleason scoring system, which assigns two numbers and a sum score. The most commonly assigned Gleason score is 3 + 3 = 6.

The classification that has been used most successfully to describe the extent of a prostate cancer is the TNM staging system. This stands for tumour, nodes, and metastases. It is an internationally recognized system which has been in use for over 50 years.

The TNM classification of prostate cancer

Tumour

The T category stands for Tumour, as assessed by a rectal examination and/or by specialized scanning such as MRI scanning.

T1   Incidental (impalpable and not detectable by ultrasound)

T1a Well-differentiated prostate cancer diagnosed at transurethral resection of the prostate (TURP) involving less than 5 per cent of the resected tissue

T1b Any tumour diagnosed at TURP which is less than well-differentiated and/or involves more than 5 per cent of resected material

T1c Impalpable prostate cancer diagnosed on TRUS-guided biopsy performed because of elevated PSA value

T2   Locally confined to the prostate

T3   Locally extensive

T4   Fixation onto, or invasion of, neighbouring organs

Nodes

This stands for lymph nodes. We have seen how tumours can invade the lymphatic system, which is a system of channels for draining fluid from tissues and organs which runs from the prostat e itself into the pelvis, and from there into the abdomen and the chest, and finally drains the fluid back into the bloodstream. There are concentrations of lymphatic tissue called lymph nodes along the channels. These may be likened to sentry points along the highway. The body's killer white blood cells reside in the lymph nodes, and sometimes the tumour can be successfully destroyed by the immune system. However, tumours can be identified in the nodes and the nodes are assessed in the following way.

N0 No regional lymph node metastasis

N1 Metastasis in single regional lymph node, <2 cm in largest dimension

N2 Metastasis in single regional lymph node, >2 cm but <5 cm in largest dimension

N3 Metastasis in regional lymph node, >5cm in largest dimension

It is possible to remove these lymph nodes surgically and this may be done as part of a radical prostatectomy operation. In some cases this can cure the patient.

Metastasis

Spread of cancer to other parts of the body, either distant lymph nodes or other organs, is classified under the M category. Metastasis particularly occurs in bones, as noted in Chapter 1, but less commonly prostate cancer can spread to other organs, such as the liver. Metastasis is classified as follows.

M0   No distant metastasis

M1   Distant metastasis

M1a Metastasis in non-regional lymph nodes

M1b Metastasis in bone

M1c Metastasis at other site

How do medical images show advanced a prostate cancer is?

Early cancer

Trans-rectal ultrasound scan (TRUS)

The first investigation you might have to undergo is likely to be a trans-rectal ultrasound scan (TRUS). This involves you lying on your side while the radiologist or urologist inserts a probe into your rectum. The probe uses ultrasound (high-frequency sound waves) to obtain a picture of your prostate. The principle of ultrasound is that echoes from the tissues bounce back, are detected by the probe, and are turned into pictures. For prostate ultrasound, the doctor will be looking for areas which have a reduced rather than normal echo pattern (hypoechoic areas) A spring-loaded gun is used to fire a needle into the prostate and biopsies are taken. These may be restricted to an abnormal area, but often four biopsies are taken from both lobes of the prostate—eight biopsies in all. Sometimes more biopsies than this are taken, as many as 12 or even 14.

This may be uncomfortable but is not as painful as you might expect, and in many cases a local anaesthetic is given before the biopsies are taken. The biopsies are then sent for examination at the pathology laboratory.

In early cancer, patients may also be sent for a CT scan or an MRI scan.

◆   **CT (computed tomography) scan** For this X-ray technique you lie on your back on a couch, and pictures, taken in many different directions, are assembled by a computer which then reconstructs an image as if a cross-section of your body had been taken.

- **MRI (magnetic resonance imaging) scan** This technique uses a strong magnetic field and radio waves, rather than X-rays, and is believed to be safer and more accurate. MRI scans are noisy, and you may be given earplugs to wear. Also, as the ring through which the couch passes is narrower and longer, some people find the experience claustrophobic. As with CT, the images are of cross-sections in various planes of the body, and are often highly detailed.

Less often, other specialist scans are done, such as PET (positron emission tomography), but this is not yet a routine scan in all centres.

The presence of spread outside into bone is found in two main ways.

- Prostate cancer seems to spread preferentially to the bones, particularly of the spine and pelvis. These secondaries, or metastases, show up as denser areas on X-ray pictures and an ordinary X-ray is sometimes a good way of showing up this type of disease.

- An additional, more sensitive, method is a bone scan. This is carried out by injecting a radioactive isotope, which goes particularly to the bones, and can be shown up by scanning all the bones after a short period of time. The radioactivity does not last long and you are perfectly safe to mix with people in company after two days.

In patients with an early-stage cancer and a PSA of less than 10, the bone scan is often omitted because the chances of it showing anything are very small.

How do we measure how aggressive a prostate cancer is?

When a biopsy is taken, a specialist pathologist looks at the tissue. He or she is skilled in looking at prostate tissue under a microscope and diagnosing a range of prostate disorders—not just cancer. If a diagnosis of prostate cancer is made, an important question is whether or not it is an aggressive cancer. While the methods for looking at this are not perfect, the usual measure of the degree of aggression is the Gleason grading system, named after the man who first described it.

The pathologist looks at the most predominant pattern and then at the next most predominant pattern and adds the two grades together to obtain a score, e.g. Gleason 3+4 = 7.

Table 2.1 Gleason grading system

Cancerous tissue pattern		Gleason grade
Non aggressive tumour	Closely packed, well-defined glands within the prostate	1
	Less uniformly shaped glands	2
	Irregular glands of variable size	3
	A mass of fused glands	4
Aggressive tumour	Few, or no, visible glands; very little difference between them	5

The final figure is a sum score and is known to relate to survival—the higher the number the shorter the survival might be. On its own, this may not give the whole story but it may help a patient to decide whether or not to have aggressive treatment. A sum score of less than 6 implies a particularly unaggressive looking tumour, while a score of more than 6, especially a score of 8–10, implies an aggressive tumour. More recently, it has become recognized that some prostate cancers have a third, or tertiary grade, pattern, and where this is present it is also recorded.

Note: Pathologists will not use a grade of less than 3 now on TRUS biopsies, and because of the small amount of tissue, usually merely double the score of 3 to give a sum score of 6.

PSA

PSA stands for prostate-specific antigen. This is a protein which is detected in the bloodstream of almost all adult men. The protein has a role in adjusting the stickiness of semen.

As men age, their prostates become bigger. This tends to make the level of PSA rise. In addition, more of the PSA 'leaks' into the bloodstream as we become older. PSA measures activity in prostate tissue. It has been found that various conditions are associated with an increase of PSA above normal levels (Table 2.2). PSA increases with age, and normal levels have been calculated for each age group.

Patients with prostate cancer usually have an increase in PSA.

The PSA level can be a useful method of determining response to treatment, whether after surgery to remove the prostate(radical prostatectomy) or after hormonal treatment in more advanced cancers.

Table 2.2 Conditions or activities causing change in PSA

Result	Condition or activity causing change in PSA
Rise	Prostate cancer
Rise	Benign prostatic hyperplasia
Rise	Prostate biopsy
Rise	Prostatitis (usually caused by infection)
Rise	Prostate manipulation (i.e. DRE or TRUS)
Rise	Cycling!
Decrease	Hormone therapy
Decrease	Prostatectomy (removal of prostate)
Variable	Sex
Variable	Exercise

DRE, digital rectal examination.

After radical prostatectomy, the PSA should fall to zero.

Prostate cancer symptoms

There are generally no symptoms associated with early prostate cancer. However, if and when they appear, the symptoms of prostate cancer and BPH are very similar. These tend to involve problems with 'the waterworks'. Patients may experience:

- difficulty or pain when passing urine

- the need to pass urine more often (frequency)

- broken sleep due to increased visits to pass urine

- waiting for long periods before the urine flows (hesitancy)

- the feeling that the bladder has not emptied fully.

These symptoms are sometimes associated with early disease and can be the first signs of prostate enlargement. Quite often, men with prostate cancer who have such symptoms have both BPH and prostate cancer, and their symptoms are actually due to the BPH and not the prostate cancer. Other symptoms, which can be associated with later-stage disease, are:

- blood in the urine (unusual)

- pain in the pelvis or loins

- blood in the sperm (very rare)

- general bone pain

- weight loss.

All of these symptoms should be reported to your doctor so that they can be investigated, although they may be caused by something other than prostate cancer.

Questions to ask your doctor

General

Do you think that I may have a problem with my prostate?

What are the advantages and disadvantages of having a PSA test?

If you find prostate cancer, what is the next step?

After you have your test results

My PSA blood test result is raised. How high is the result and what could this mean?

How certain can you be that I have prostate cancer and not another prostate condition?

What can you tell me about the cancer (size, position, speed, and growth)?

Which do you feel would be the most suitable treatment for me and why?

If I choose to be treated, will the treatment relieve my symptoms?

What are the side effects of the treatment and how might they affect my lifestyle?

3

Risks and benefits of screening and radical treatment—a guide

> ### 🡒 Key points
>
> ◆ There are many risks and benefits of treatment of prostate cancer which can make the decision process difficult
>
> ◆ Some patients with prostate cancer are treated unnecessarily, as it can be a harmless illness
>
> ◆ Screening is not totally reliable as a means of detecting prostate cancer

Almost anything in life has associated risks. It is not perhaps surprising that parachuting in the USA carries a risk 19 000 times that of playing Association Football in England and Wales. Climbing in England and Wales carries 130 times the risk of playing football. Surgical anaesthesia in England in 1986 had a risk of death of 5.4 cases per million operations.

One of the most difficult aspects of prostate cancer is that the decision-making process may be presented to you as a 'risks versus benefits' equation. This is a difficult concept, particularly when many of the risks seem far away if you are one of the lucky ones who have no symptoms whatsoever. It is also a difficult subject for doctors and nurses to convey well, and in this section we attempt to represent some of the issues in a graphical manner.

We are beginning to get some idea of how many prostate cancers are treated unnecessarily if they are discovered by testing for PSA in men who are otherwise well. This has come from the recent European screening study which suggests that, for every man whose prostate cancer needed treatment, another 47 received treatment that they did not need (Figure 3.1). On the other hand,

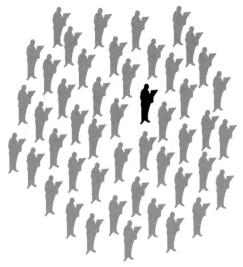

Figure 3.1 For every man whose prostate cancer needed treatment, another 47 received treatment that they did not need.

we have evidence from a large study conducted in Sweden that treatment does actually cure some men who have prostate cancer localized to the prostate gland itself. Conversely, some men with aggressive prostate cancer will eventually die from their disease despite the best efforts of today's treatments. For you as an individual, and for your doctors, there is a dilemma.

The famous urologist Walt Whitmore summed up the dilemma thus:

Is a cure possible in patients in whom it might be necessary?

Is a cure necessary in patients in whom it might be possible?

It is believed that up to 80 per cent of *all* men develop prostate cancer by the age of 80. Nothing like this number of men suffer harm from their cancer, implying that in most men prostate cancer is a harmless illness.

The estimate of 1 in 48 (even if it is accurate) is at best an overall figure, which can be of limited value for you, as an individual patient. To illustrate this, let us consider a patient who is found to have a small cancer, which is not visible or palpable (i.e. the prostate gland feels normal), who has a PSA in the normal range for his age, and whose Gleason sum score (see Chapter 2) is only 3.

19

His chances of 'significant' disease might be 1 in 100 rather than 1 in 48, which would look pictorially as shown in Figure 3.2. Even this estimate, which is also highly theoretical, takes no account of the patient's age. The younger a patient, the greater the chances his prostate cancer may have to cause him harm. For a patient aged 50, the lifetime chance of the above tumour causing harm might be 1 in 20, whereas the same tumour in a patient aged 80 might have a lifetime chance of causing harm of only 1 in 200.

Now, let us consider a tumour that is palpable (can be felt on examination), but is confined to the prostate gland. It has a Gleason sum score of 8. This tumour is much more likely to cause harm at all ages, although in a younger patient it is perhaps particularly likely to have the opportunity to do so (say, at any time over the next 30 years). The risks of such a tumour, if untreated, causing harm to a man aged 50 at some stage in his lifetime might be 2 in 3. In a man aged 80, destined to live for another 5 years, it might be 1 in 5. These risks could be represented pictorially in Figure 3.3.

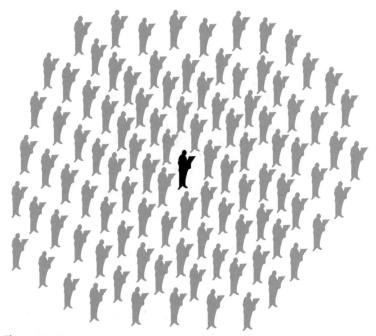

Figure 3.2 One man in 100 has a 'significant' or harmful prostate cancer, although the cancers look the same in all 100 men.

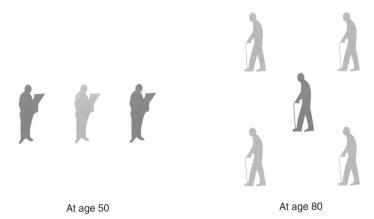

At age 50   At age 80

Figure 3.3 The risk from a cancer getting worse (disease progression) also depends on a person's age. In this example, a man with a significanr prostate cancer, disgnosed at age 50, has a 2 in 3 lifetime risk of it progressing.

Note that even in this hypothetical situation, where we have assumed that we actually know the risks (and, again, it is emphasized that we *do not*), we cannot predict with certainty what *will* happen to an individual patient, only what *might* happen. However, although the figures themselves are hypothetical, the general ranking of risk is accurate. In other words, an untreated tumour is least likely to cause harm if it is well differentiated, impalpable, associated with a low PSA, and presents in an elderly man. An untreated tumour is most likely to cause harm if it is poorly differentiated, palpable, and associated with a high PSA in a young man. Many tumours fall into the middle of these extremes—for example, a moderately differentiated tumour which is visible on scans but not palpable and is associated with a mildly elevated PSA in a man aged 62.

All these considerations make the issues of screening and treatment more complex than might have appeared at first sight. However, to complicate the situation further, we must return to our initial assumption—that is, that if a cancer were present, it would be detected. Unfortunately, this is not always the case. Although a combination of PSA, rectal examination, and TRUS is a highly sensitive means of detecting a prostate cancer, these techniques are far from perfect, and some patients with significant cancers may be wrongly labelled as being 'all clear'. Other patients, who do not have cancer, can have a scare when screening tests suggest that they do, until they are later proved to be 'all clear'.

In summary:

* Screening is not perfect. It might unnecessarily scare a man who actually does not have prostate cancer.

* Treatment is not perfect. It might cause harm to a man whose prostate cancer would not have caused him harm.

* Equally, treatment will cure some patients, although as yet we do not have a reliable way of identifying which men they are.

* Treatment may prevent disease progression, which in itself could be beneficial, irrespective of whether or not it also cures people.

* Screening is not perfect. It might wrongly reassure a man who actually does have prostate cancer, but in whom it is not detected.

* If a prostate cancer is discovered, it is impossible to predict what *will* happen to the patient. It is a little easier to guess as to how likely a cancer, if untreated, *might* cause a man harm at some time during his lifetime, but our weighing of the risks is based on crude estimates, not facts.

* In assessing the risks to an individual, doctors would need to consider his age, the size of the tumour, its grade (Gleason sum score), and his PSA level.

This discussion is not an argument against screening or radical treatment. The European Randomized Trial of Screening for Prostate Cancer has been an incredibly important advance, and for the first time gives us some estimates of what the real benefits of PSA screening might be. However, more information will come from this, and other trials, in the future. For you, as a patient, the evidence that we have suggests that there are no 'rights' or 'wrongs'. Whether or not you should undergo PSA testing, if you have no symptoms, is a personal choice, and even in the USA, where regular PSA screening has been the norm for over a decade, the official advice has been watered down. The dilemma of whether or not to be screened is particularly relevant when the risks of 'radical' treatment (which really just means 'curative' treatment, usually by radical prostatectomy or radical radiotherapy) are considered, and these are discussed in Chapter 4.

4

Treatment and management options

➜ Key points

◆ For the majority of men diagnosed with prostate cancer, there will be no signs of the cancer anywhere other than in the prostate gland.

◆ The choice of treatment options is bewildering, not least because it is wrapped up in two questions:

Should I have treatment immediately, or can this be delayed until/unless my prostate cancer shows signs of getting worse?

If I have treatment now, what treatment should I have?

◆ Treatment options include various types of radiotherapy, and surgery

General introduction—a guide to choice of treatment

In this chapter we consider the different ways of treating the prostate gland. Deciding which of these options is the most appropriate can be one of the most difficult aspects of managing prostate cancer, and is often bewildering for doctor and patient alike. The reason for this difficulty is simple—*we do not know the best treatment for prostate cancer*. For a number of reasons, not the least of which may be technical, not every patient is suitable for every form of treatment. This important aspect is something that you should discuss with the specialist.

The 'success rate' after radical treatment depends on a complex and wide-ranging number of variables. It varies hugely between patients, and therefore, deliberately, treatment results are not given here. Additionally, the lack of high-quality randomized trials comparing treatments means that their respective 'success' rates are difficult to gauge.

Table 4.1 Patient classification

Low risk	PSA less than 10, Gleason 2–6, and stage T1–T2a
Intermediate risk	PSA 10–20, Gleason 7, or stage T2b–T2c
High risk	PSA over 20, Gleason 8–10, or stage T3–T4

In recent years, there has been a growing tendency to classify patients into 'prognostic groups', in other words, to group them according to the various factors that affect their outcome in terms of prostate cancer. Broadly, these are tumour stage (TNM category), Gleason score, and PSA level. Using these variables, patients are classified into 'low-risk', 'intermediate-risk', and 'high-risk' categories (Table 4.1). Patients whose general health and life expectancy are otherwise good need to consider two questions, which they should discuss with their specialists:

1. Should I have treatment now or defer treatment until/unless my prostate cancer shows some evidence of getting worse (progressing)?

2. If I am going to have treatment now, what form should it take? The two major alternatives are surgery and radiotherapy (both are available in several forms). There are other options, such as cryotherapy and high-frequency ultrasound (HIFU), which do not yet have the same weight of experience or evidence to back them up, and which should only be performed in highly specialized centres.

Active monitoring or active surveillance

Active monitoring in early disease

Active monitoring is also known as surveillance therapy, expectant management, or observation. Essentially, active monitoring implies that the patient has initially decided with his doctor to avoid immediate active treatment, but to monitor the disease by estimating the PSA at several monthly intervals and tracking it.

In any other cancer, this would seem a strange concept. The reasons why active monitoring may be sensible in some patients are, first, that we know that not all cancers will progress during the patient's lifetime to cause him trouble, and, secondly, that all the treatments, descriptions of which follow, have side effects. Sometimes it is quite possible to balance the risks of treatment versus the risks of the disease getting worse (progressing).

We know that certain patients with early-stage cancers have at least an 80 per cent chance that their disease will not progress. Active monitoring does not imply a lack of treatment, but rather a deferral of treatment unless it appears to be necessary. To date, the evidence suggests that survival rates following this policy are no worse than they are in patients who opt for immediate treatment. Patients who opt for active monitoring, and whose disease does not progress, reap the obvious benefit that they have avoided treatment—hence they have avoided treatment side effects—at no cost to their health. Even patients who opt for active monitoring but whose disease does progress, resulting in the need for treatment, do not appear to have been disadvantaged by the delay in their treatment. Having said this, there are no published randomized trials which compare active monitoring with immediate surgery or radiotherapy, although two such trials are in progress (ProtecT and ProSTART). The evidence comes from centres with extensive experience of active monitoring, most notably the Princess Margaret Hospital in Toronto and the Royal Marsden Hospital in London.

The exact procedure for active monitoring varies somewhat from centre to centre, but generally involves a PSA test every few months—probably around three-monthly to begin with, but maybe extending to longer intervals with time. Often this is combined with a digital rectal examination, and a repeat transrectal ultrasound and prostate biopsy may be performed in some centres, although this is not universal.

 Patient perspective

John is a 77-year-old retired engineer. He had a prostate cancer diagnosed 8 years ago, at which time his PSA was 4.5. He decided to opt for active monitoring, which began with three-monthly visits and PSA tests, and he is now being seen six-monthly. His PSA has gone up and down during this time, but the highest reading was 6.2. His latest result is 4.9, and he continues on active monitoring.

John says 'I am pleased that I went for this option; I was particularly concerned with the side effects of treatment, so when my doctor suggested that my prostate cancer might be very slow growing, this seemed like a sensible thing to do at my age. It can be stressful waiting for the results of a PSA test, and especially when it has gone up a bit and the doctors have to decide what to do. However, I have managed to avoid an operation or radiotherapy so far, which is a good outcome for me.'

Active monitoring after failure of primary therapy

Unfortunately, after a radical prostatectomy, a number of patients may find that they have what is called 'margin-positive disease'. Although this is disappointing, 50 per cent of these patients do not appear to progress and so there is an argument for managing this situation by active monitoring. However, there are now three randomized trials which compare immediate radiotherapy to the area of the pelvis where the prostate was with deferred treatment, all of which suggest that the risk of disease progression is significantly reduced by radiotherapy. However, two questions remain. The first is whether radiotherapy should be given alone, or whether it should be combined with hormone therapy (and if so, for how long the hormone therapy should last). The second question is whether radiotherapy should be given immediately or deferred—the same question that the three randomized trials answered—and this question is quite deliberately being asked again because of one highly important technological advance, i.e. it is possible to detect PSA in the blood with 100 times the sensitivity that was available with the PSA tests at the time that these trials first began. This means that, in theory, it might be possible to defer so-called 'salvage' radiotherapy until/unless the PSA shows definite sings of rising, but is still at extremely low levels, at a time when the amount of cancer present would be microscopically small. Such an approach would allow the 50 per cent of patients in this situation, who never progressed, to avoid salvage radiotherapy altogether. This approach, together with the need for and duration of hormone therapy, is currently being tested in the Medical Research Council 'RADICALS' trial.

Occasionally patients will fail after radiotherapy (external beam or brachytherapy). The levels of PSA may be very low initially and the radiotherapist will wish to look at the doubling time of the PSA, as well as the absolute levels. Some patients whose PSA recurs after surgery or radiotherapy may have such a slow doubling time that they will never come to harm from their prostate cancer. In terms of active monitoring, it is important to remember that it is unfortunate if a patient has treatment, with a lot of side effects, without benefit. Many patients who 'fail' their first treatment will still never die of their prostate cancer.

Watchful waiting in advanced disease

In patients with advanced disease who have no symptoms, a situation which is not uncommon, there is an argument for deferring treatment until the patient has symptoms. However, with the development of newer anti-androgens and luteinizing hormone-releasing hormone (LHRH) analogues, the toxicity is very much less. Nonetheless, all these drug treatments carry some risk.

There are a number of other reasons why patients may wish to have earlier treatment. Some patients cannot bear the thought that their cancer is not being confronted. There is a risk that the bulk of disease will increase and it will become more difficult for the tumour to be controlled. There is the very real risk that the patient may develop side effects and spinal problems, because of a collapse of bones, with secondary disease. There is the possibility that the untreated prostate cancer may become less hormone sensitive is it develops, although the evidence for this is much less. Local progression of prostate cancer may require the patient to have an operation on his prostate because of urinary blockage.

There is a feeling that, in advanced disease, deferred treatment may reduce survival and there is also a risk that some patients could die from prostate cancer without receiving treatment if not monitored carefully.

A large trial performed by the Medical Research Council appeared to show a marginal improvement in survival, but undoubtedly a lower risk of complications. However, the differences were not considerable, and it is interesting to note that 27 patients receiving immediate treatment died from cancer of other organs, quite unrelated to their prostate cancer. The risk of death from heart disease and strokes appeared to be similar in both groups.

Radiotherapy

Introduction

Radical radiotherapy is reserved for men whose disease appears possible to eradicate completely, in the hope that this will cure the patient. Radiotherapy (or X-ray therapy) is a treatment which uses high-energy X-rays to kill cancer cells. It has been known for a long time that X-rays damage cells—both normal cells and cancer cells. However, cancer cells have a reduced ability to repair X-ray-induced damage, and this is the basis of radiotherapy. Treatment is given in such a way that normal cells are able to recover, whereas cancer cells are not. There are two general methods for delivering radiotherapy:

- external beam radiotherapy, in which the patient lies on a couch and X-rays are directed from a machine (a linear accelerator, or Linac) onto the pelvis, targeted at the prostate gland;

- brachytherapy, in which radioactive seeds, which emit X-rays, are implanted into the prostate gland, usually under a general anaesthetic and in the operating theatre.

These are considered here in turn.

External beam radiotherapy

This is the most common form of radiotherapy. Among its advantages are that it can be given as an outpatient treatment, and that most patients are able to tolerate it without undue side effects. In order to succeed, the treatment has to be custom designed for each patient to ensure that a high dose of X-rays can be given to the prostate gland, while as low a dose as possible is given to the surrounding tissues. The treatment planning to achieve this usually involves a CT or MRI scan, which gives a cross-sectional image of the prostate and surrounding tissues, and provides information that the radiotherapist can feed directly into the planning computer (Figure 4.1). This is why a planning scan may be needed, even if the patient has already had a previous CT or MRI scan. The radiotherapy physicist can then use a planning computer to work out the best X-ray beam size and arrangement. Typically, a patient, lying on his back on a treatment couch, is treated with the machine directing the X-ray beam at him from several different directions, typically between four and eight. Each treatment takes a few minutes; indeed, it takes longer to ensure that a patient is in the correct position (to within millimetres) than it does to administer the treatment itself. This is repeated, on a daily basis

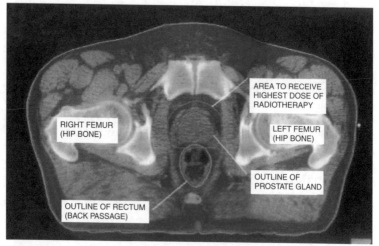

Figure 4.1 The appearance of the prostate gland as viewed in the course of radiotherapy planning. Two outlines have been drawn using the planning computer. One encircles the prostate gland itself and the other, generated by the computer, adds a margin of 1 cm to this, in all directions except behind the prostate, where the margin is reduced to 5 mm to minimize the amount of the rectum in the radiotherapy field.

(usually excluding weekends), for 4–8 weeks (depending on the exact details of the technique, which vary between hospitals).

New radiotherapy technology—conformal therapy

Conventionally, radiotherapy planning makes use of two-dimensional images from a CT scan, i.e. pictures of the body in cross-section. A three-dimensional image of the prostate, tumour, and surrounding tissues can be built up from these pictures. However, until very recently, a limitation of radiotherapy was that the head of a linear accelerator (the part from which the X-rays emerge into the open air) was rectangular. Its jaws could move to give X-ray beams of different sizes, but they would only be square or rectangular. Thus the area of the body which received the highest dose would be cylindrical in shape; however, tumours, prostates, and normal parts of the body are not cylindrical but irregular in shape.

Conformal radiotherapy uses an X-ray head which produces a beam which is not only irregular in shape, but can also be made into any shape that the therapist may desire. This is done by means of a so-called multileaf collimator, which divides the jaws into a series of 'mini-jaws' that can be opened and shut independently of each other and to an independent extent. The result is that treatment can be better tailored to an individual's shape and size, plus the position and shape of the prostate/tumour. Although this has been used primarily as a way of reducing the side effects of radiotherapy, it could also be a means whereby a higher dose of radiation can be given, at the cost of a similar rate of side effects compared with conventional treatment, but with a higher chance of tumour control. This possibility is currently being investigated in a UK clinical trial.

This can reduce side effects, but does not abolish them. Patients undergoing radiotherapy feel nothing at all while the machine is switched on. However, side effects do occur over the whole 4–8-week course of treatment, and these need to be discussed. The side effects of radiotherapy can be divided into acute side effects (those that occur during and immediately after the individual's radiotherapy) and late side effects (those that occur months or even years after the radiotherapy has been completed).

Intensity-modulated radiotherapy (IMRT)

This is a further development of the conformal approach, which makes use of the ability of modern Linacs to vary the position of their multileaf collimators dynamically while the treatment is in progress. This is useful where the desired treatment area would be concave, even in part, a challenge which pure conformal therapy cannot rise to. For many prostate cancer patients, the desired treatment area will be entirely convex, and IMRT may not offer them any particular advantages.

Image-guided radiotherapy (IGRT)

This refinement is becoming more widely available in prostate cancer treatments. It allows images to be taken when the patient is lying on the Linac couch and any corrections for movement to be made (for example of the prostate itself which, although formerly thought to be static in position, can actually move), so increasing the accuracy of the treatment delivery even further (it is already possible to deliver radiotherapy with millimetre acuracy).

Acute side effects

The urethra, which carries urine out of the bladder, passes right through the centre of the prostate gland. Inflammation of the urethra and bladder during a course of radiotherapy causes discomfort when passing urine, and more frequent passage of urine. Because the prostate gland is so closely associated with the rectum (back passage), radiotherapy to the prostate gland inevitably involves giving a certain dose of radiation to the rectum. This results in a degree of inflammation, which manifests itself as diarrhoea, perhaps even with the passage of a small amount of blood. These side effects usually start after about 2 weeks of radiotherapy, and can worsen over the remaining period. Generally, they settle around 4–6 weeks after the end of the course of treatment. In addition, patients may be more tired than usual during radiotherapy. Diarrhoea can be managed with medication or modification of diet, and urinary problems can be managed with fluids and sometimes antibiotics.

Long-term side effects

Uncommonly, acute side effects either fail to settle or, cruelly, settle initially and then return after 6 months to 2 years. It is uncommomn for such side effects to be significant enough to interfere with a man's life; this occurs in 1–5 per cent of patients. However, it is worrying for those patients in whom it occurs, as such side effects may be permanent. They respond to some degree to other treatments, but may not go away completely. In addition, 45 per cent or more of men who are potent before radiotherapy may become impotent by 5 years after treatment. Incontinence following external beam radiotherapy is rare except in men who have had a previous TURP.

Brachytherapy in prostate cancer

Modern brachytherapy is a two-stage procedure. In the first stage the prostatic volume is measured using transrectal ultrasound, and the data obtained are used to plan the number and positioning of radioactive sources in an attempt to deliver a homogeneous dose of radiation to the prostate. The second stage involves inserting the sources into the pre-planned position through a needle under general anaesthetic. Usually, these needles are inserted through the perineal skin between the legs. Implants can be either removed or left in permanently; in the UK most are permanent. Brachytherapy should theoretically have an advantage in terms of damage to adjacent structures, such as the rectum and the nerves that were alongside the prostate. The disadvantage is that the area extending more than 3–4 mm outside the prostate capsule will not be irradiated, so any stray cancer cells present may not be treated. Not every patient is suitable for brachytherapy; for example, some centres will not use it to treat patients who have undergone a previous TURP. Similarly, some patients who have a large prostate, even when the enlargement is due to benign disease and not to their prostate cancer, may be unsuitable for brachytherapy, as may patients with a large cancer in the prostate gland or those with a high Gleason grade.

Complications

Patients can develop significant urinary symptoms (see above) following prostate brachytherapy. In some series, 4–8 per cent of patients required catheterization or cystoscopy in the weeks following brachytherapy. Bowel complications occur in less than 2 per cent of patients receiving implants as the sole treatment, and incontinence occurs in up to 1 per cent.

 Patient perspective

It is now nearly 3 years since my radiotherapy. Generally speaking, I have no ill-effects; I do notice though that, whereas I used to open my bowels once a day, I now tend to go twice a day. My doctor tells me that it is a result of the radiotherapy, but it doesn't bother me now that I know what it is.

Surgery

Surgical removal of a cancer is a well-established treatment for many types of cancer. In the case of prostate cancer, the operation removes the entire prostate and not just the cancer. It must be stressed that a transurethral resection of the prostate (TURP) does not do this; it merely removes the central 'core' of the prostate. Prostate cancers occur in other regions of the prostate, and there may be several separate tumours within the prostate gland. There are two main disadvantages of surgery: first, incontinence (being unable to control the flow of urine), and, secondly, loss of sexual potency. In 1982, Patrick Walsh of the

Johns Hopkins University, Baltimore, USA, developed a technique of removing the prostate but sparing the nerves which control erections. However, it must be emphasized that not every patient is suitable for this approach, although for suitable patients there is an operation where sexual ability is not necessarily lost.

Radical surgery is reserved for men for whom it appears possible to remove the disease completely, in the hope that this will cure the patient. It is also important that they will live long enough to benefit from any cure. This means that a patient must have a life expectancy of at least 10 years before radical surgery is considered. The age and general health of the patient are also important. Age itself is not a bar to treatment, but the presence of other serious medical conditions can make surgery hazardous.

The operation

It is usual for surgery to be postponed for about 8 weeks after a needle biopsy of the prostate and for 12 weeks after a TURP (see later). In North America and certain European countries, the patient may be given the opportunity to donate two or three units of blood, which can be transfused back into him if required. This is called autologous blood transfusion. Patients are usually advised to avoid taking aspirin and non-steroidal anti-inflammatory drugs, which interfere with the function of blood clotting. The anaesthetist will discuss the type of anaesthetic, which may be a general or spinal anaesthetic.

The incision is made from just above the pubic bone to the umbilicus (tummy button). The prostate is then removed through the abdomen and the remaining bladder is joined to the end of the urethra. The patient is normally allowed a clear liquid diet on the first postoperative day, building up to a regular diet on the third day. There may be suction drains coming from separate areas of the abdomen and these are removed when they stop discharging.

A catheter will have been placed in the bladder and the patient goes home with the catheter in position, returning 3 weeks after the procedure for removal.

Complications

The death rate is low—of the order of 0.2 per cent. Complications at operation are bleeding, damage to the obturator nerve (supplying muscles in the leg), injury to the rectum, and occasionally injury to the ureter.

Fewer than 10 per cent of men are significantly incontinent after surgery. However, the figure may be higher than this; figures of 25–30 per cent are reported, although most commonly this is minor and may improve. Patients over

65 appear to have a greater risk of incontinence. Continence should return in most men by 12 months, with over half achieving continence within 3 months. If incontinence continues, treatments are available to deal with this.

Where the nerve bundles have been preserved, potency should return in at least 50 per cent of men. Sildenafil (Viagra) or apomorphine (Uprima) are effective in some patients where potency has not been achieved (see Chapter 12).

The perineal operation

This operation, although less popular worldwide, is achieving greater popularity. It is performed in the crutch, below the scrotum, and does not require a large cut on the abdomen. Blood loss is much less and patients return home sooner. There is debate as to whether it preserves the nerves as well as the open operation. Continence rates appear to be similar to those of the open operation, as is the control of cancer.

 Patient perspective

I've been pretty good since my surgery. My erections are not so good, but I am taking Viagra. My control of urine is pretty good. I sometimes wear a pad while I am playing golf, as I used to get a small dribble when I took a swing, but to be honest, it is more a precaution than anything else.

5

Screening

 Key points

- Screening for prostate cancer is still a controversial issue as there are many advantages and disadvantages

- PSA screening involves a blood test, and can lead to subsequent complicated and often unpleasant tests. There is little point in having a PSA test done unless you are prepared to undergo the next steps if it is found to be raised.

- There is ongoing research into the best way to screen for and detect prostate cancer

 Should I be screened for prostate cancer?

If you are a healthy man wondering what to do if offered a PSA test, then this chapter can help.

Why is screening for prostate cancer so controversial? To many people, it seems obvious that, in order to cure more men of prostate cancer, screening should enable a diagnosis to be made at the earliest possible stage and should be done as a matter of course. Despite this, the reluctance of the UK government to institute a screening programme seems implacable. To understand the scientific, as opposed to the political, reasons behind this, we must look at both the advantages and the disadvantages of prostate cancer screening.

Before doing this, we briefly consider what screening involves. The most common practice is to use a blood test for PSA (prostate-specific antigen, see

Chapter 1). In patients whose PSA level is elevated, further tests are performed. This will involve a consultation with a specialist, usually a urologist. He will perform a rectal examination (see Chapter 1) and subsequently an ultrasound test, which is carried out using a probe inserted into the rectum. This may or may not identify an abnormality in the prostate. In either event, it will be necessary to biopsy the prostate gland, which is carried out with a needle that passes through the rectum and into the gland. If the ultrasound identifies an abnormality, it will be biopsied, but if no abnormality is seen, the prostate will need to be biopsied 'blindly'. Usually, six or eight biopsy samples are taken (from the upper, middle, and lower part of the gland on each side). It may be that, in the future, even more samples will be taken. This can be an unpleasant procedure, and a proportion of men develop an infection following this (although treating all patients who have a biopsy with antibiotics reduces this). If the biopsy shows evidence of prostate cancer, the treatment options then need to be discussed. If the biopsy does not show prostate cancer, there are a number of options for the next step, which very much depend on the overall picture. It may be necessary to repeat the transrectal ultrasound scan and biopsy in the future. This would particularly be the case if the biopsy showed changes that in themselves were not cancerous, but which are known to precede cancer in some men (this is prostatic intra-epithelial neoplasia, or PIN).

It may be clear by now that the blood test for PSA, the initial test in the screening process, is the simplest one to undertake (from both the patient's and the doctor's point of view). The subsequent tests are more complicated and more unpleasant. They are also not perfect, in the sense that they may not give a definitive answer to the question 'Have I got prostate cancer?' or may even give the wrong answer. This is part of the reason for the controversy. Another is that some men, although they do not have definite evidence of prostate cancer, may have some evidence of other changes in the prostate, for example PIN. PIN is not cancer, but it may result in men having to have repeat biopsies to check whether or not they are developing cancer.

Let us now consider the **advantages** and **disadvantages** of screening. The advantages are:

- that it may allow a cure of an otherwise fatal disease

- that, by identifying a cancer at an early stage, treatment might be more straightforward than if it had been discovered later

- that introducing a screening service would also introduce well-organized networks of specialists involved in treating prostate cancer.

> **?** These are pretty big advantages, especially the first, so why the controversy?

The first disadvantage of screening is that, although we now believe that screening based on PSA does reduce deaths from prostate cancer, the true costs of this, in terms of both money and the risks of harm to men who are screened, seem to be high. This sounds like a strange statement, so let us examine it further.

Leaving aside the purely financial costs of screening all men using PSA (estimated by one expert at £1.3 billion per year in the UK), there is the knowledge, now certain, that screening results in 'overtreatment'; in other words, for every man whose prostate cancer needed to be detected and treated in order to save his life, many more were treated who did not need to be treated. This would not matter if the treatments themselves were easy or harmless, but they are not. As discussed in Chapter 4, treatment with surgery carries a risk of impotence and incontinence, while treatment with radiotherapy carries a risk of bowel problems. It is even possible that (extremely rarely), some men might die as a result of a treatment which they did not need in the first place.

Information from the European screening trial has suggested that, in order to save one man's life, 48 men need to be treated for prostate cancer and 1000 men need to be screened (see Figure 3.1). Of the 48 men treated, perhaps one or two will suffer significant or major side effects from their treatment, while many more will suffer from definite but less significant side effects. A second clinical trial of screening, from the USA, apparently showed no benefit whatsoever. However, part of the reason for this might be that a large number of men who were in the 'control' group (in other words, men who were not supposed to be screened for prostate cancer) actually did receive a PSA test, so this trial may not have given a fair comparison of 'PSA test' versus 'no PSA test'.

What is the way forward? There are many research avenues which are trying to refine the information that the PSA test can give us. One such method is to use a urine test called PCA3 in combination with PSA. The PCA3 test is taken by passing a urine sample after the doctor has performed a rectal examination (see Chapter 1), and so far it looks as if it might be capable of reducing the number of men who have unnecessary (and unpleasant) biopsies. In the future, there will very likely be other tests, which may be blood tests, urine tests, or both, which might result in further refinement. Another approach would be to set a higher value of PSA before a biopsy is recommended.

Despite all this, screening, at least in its present form with PSA, may not give the correct answer, or even a definitive answer. Quite apart from the stress, and the unpleasantness of the investigations when a definite answer is given, the extra psychological stress of screening in general (especially when it has to be repeated) is now known to be real, and is very well described. Finally, even when we know that a patient has prostate cancer, we may not know what the best form of treatment is, or even whether it needs treatment at all (see Chapter 4).

Will there be any more clinical trials of screening using PSA? In the UK, a study termed the ProtecT Study is identifying healthy men who are invited to undergo a combination of PSA testing plus (if they turn out to have prostate cancer) a randomized study (see Chapter 10) of active monitoring versus radical prostatectomy versus radical radiotherapy (it must be stressed that this study is limited to nine UK centres and is not nationwide). However, it will be many years before the results are known.

A special group of men who deserve mention are those with a strong family history of prostate cancer. It seems that, for these men, there may be a genetic component to the cancer which runs in the family, and it might be sensible for close relatives in such families to receive PSA screening, especially if the men in their families seem to develop prostate cancer at an early age (such as in their forties or fifties). For such men, the risks versus benefits equation might conceivably be very different to the majority of men without a strong genetic component, and the risks of treating such men unnecessarily might be much lower than the 1 in 48 figure suggests. Studies are going on at present to address this question in such high-risk men.

So, in the meantime, what do you do? There really is no 'right' or 'wrong' answer to the question 'Should I have my PSA measured?' Part of the considerations might be—if you turned out to have prostate cancer, how would you want it to be managed? By immediate treatment (e.g. with surgery or radiotherapy) or by active monitoring? How much would you value the 1 in 1000 chance that by having a PSA test, you might be cured of a prostate cancer that would otherwise kill you? And, if you do turn out to have prostate cancer, how much would you value the 1 in 48 chance that your treatment would be necessary against the possibility of side effects if it was not. For some men, the balance is in favour of having a PSA test—they would rather know than not know. If you are one of these men, then a PSA test is probably the right thing for you. For some men, the risks that they will suffer unnecessary harm outweigh the potential benefits, and for them a PSA test may not be the right thing. However, all men should keep this question under review—this is a rapidly changing field and the next few years may well see some new light shed on this very modern dilemma, and a change in policies that might reduce the figure from 1 in 48 to a more compelling one.

6

Hormone therapy

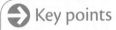 Key points

♦ Hormone therapy has been a mainstay of prostate cancer treatment for over 60 years, although many men with very early prostate cancer do not require it.

♦ It may involve short-term treatment (e.g. for a few months), as a prelude to radiotherapy, or long-term treatment (e.g. for 3 years or indefinitely).

♦ There are different forms of hormone therapy, but they all have side effects which need to be discussed with your doctor.

Prostate cancer requires the male sexual hormone, testosterone, in order to continue growing. It has been known for over 50 years that if the action of testosterone is interfered with or the tumour is deprived of testosterone, its cells will die. Testosterone deprivation (also called 'androgen deprivation' or simply 'hormone therapy') will keep a tumour under control for some time—maybe for some years. However, it usually does not completely eradicate it; rather, a state of 'détente' between the body and the tumour is reached. The most obvious means of androgen deprivation is to remove the testicles.

Hormone therapy may be used at various stages of the disease. Some patients will have hormone therapy prior to, during, and even after a course of radical radiotherapy (see Chapter 4). Hormone therapy may be used by itself in patients with locally advanced disease (see Chapter 7) or with metastatic disease.

The first effective drug treatment for prostate cancer was a compound called diethylstilboestrol (DES) or stilboestrol, which is actually a female hormone. This is an effective treatment for prostate cancer, but is less commonly used now because of its side effects, particularly heart disease, stroke, and gynaeco-mastia (enlargement of the male breast). In recent years, there has been more interest in using stilboestrol, or other forms of oestrogens, at low doses where the side effects may be far less.

Hormone therapy causes side effects similar to the menopause in women. These include hot flushes (called hot flashes in North America) and sexual problems, such that nearly all men will become impotent and lose sexual interest. In addition, some forms of hormone therapy given by tablet can cause liver problems and gynaecomastia. Gynaecomastia does not generally cause enlargement to a degree that it is noticeable to others, but if you were affected, you might notice it yourself, or be aware of it in the changing room or on the beach.

Gonadorelin (gonadotrophin or LHRH) analogues

The pituitary gland, which lies at the base of the brain, controls the production of the male sexual hormone and other hormones. It does this by releasing messenger hormones called follicle-stimulating hormone (FSH) and lutein-izing hormone (LH). Gonadorelin analogues interfere with the production of these hormones. They are given as an injection under the skin. During the initial weeks there may be actually be an increase in production of testoster-one by the testicles, and in some patients this can lead to an increased growth of the tumour, which is called 'tumour flare'. This can, for example, increase bone pain and even lead to spinal problems.

In view of this, where there is a possibility that this may occur, another drug called an anti-androgen, such as cyproterone acetate or flutamide, may be given, as a tablet, at least 3 days before the gonadorelin analogue is given. The anti-androgen is normally continued for up to 3 weeks after the first injection.

Recently, a new class of drugs called LHRH antagonists, which do not need the extra treatment with the anti-androgen, have been discovered.

Various preparations of gonadorelin

These all have their advantages and disadvantages. In the UK, the most commonly prescribed forms are goserelin and leuprorelin.

Buserelin

This is given by an injection under the skin in the abdomen every 8 hours and then by nasal spray—one spray into each nostril six times daily.

Suprefact

This is given by an injection under the skin in the abdomen every 8 hours and then by nasal spray—one spray into each nostril six times daily.

Goserelin (Zoladex)

This is given by injection every 28 days. There is also a preparation available (Zoladex LA) which is given every 12 weeks.

Leuprorelin acetate

This is available as a subcutaneous injection, given either every 4 weeks or every 3 months. A long-acting preparation may be given every 12 weeks.

Decapeptyl

This is given by intramuscular injection every 4 weeks.

Degarelix

This is a LHRH antagonist, given by injection under the skin every 28 days.

Anti-androgens

There are three main anti-androgens, which act in a way different from the gonadorelins. They interfere with the action of testosterone, rather than reducing its levels. Because they act in this way, they can be given to cover the period of potential flare when gonadorelins are started.

Cyproterone acetate (Cyprostat, Androcur)

This drug, usually given as 300 mg in two to three divided doses daily, can damage the liver directly, and liver function tests are required before treatment. It is not normally recommended for long-term treatment of prostate cancer because of the reported side effects.

Flutamide

This causes gynaecomastia (enlargement of the male breast) and can also cause diarrhoea and various other abdominal symptoms. It can also damage the liver. It is occasionally used in patients where they wish to preserve sexual function. It is not clear whether it is quite as effective as the other agents in controlling cancer, but any differences are probably small. Patients often decide on this drug after discussion.

Bicalutamide (Casodex)

This is given as 150 mg once daily, by tablet. Side effects include hot flushes and gynaecomastia. It may preserve sexual interest more than other drugs, but is not usually used alone for patients with metastases, unless they are part of a drug trial.

Coping with side effects

You should be reassured that if you are having hormonal treatment, it will not make you become effeminate. You will not look like a woman, even if oestrogens are used. Although beard growth may be slowed up, and there may be some loss of body hair, none of these treatments will cause hair loss on the head. To those not 'in the know', a patient on hormone therapy will look completely normal. They should also be reassured that their voice will not change.

Hot flushes

Hot flushes can vary from being trivial to quite disabling. It is rare that treatment has to be discontinued. These symptoms are very similar to those that happen to women when they are going through the change of life. Where flushes are troublesome, they can easily be treated with a small dose of cyproterone acetate, by tablet, or by using a drug called Provera (medroxyprogesterone acetate).

Other side effects of hormone therapy

Recently, there a lot more information has become available about other side effects of hormone therapy, generally when it is given for a long time. You should be aware of these side effects, and you may wish to discuss them with your doctor.

It appears that men who are on hormone therapy are more likely than the average to suffer from heart attacks, strokes, or diabetes, perhaps accompanied by high blood pressure. These illnesses are common in the general population, and the risks are not, in themselves, a reason not to have hormone therapy, as the increase in risk is relatively small. Bear in mind that it took studies of tens of thousands of patients to detect these risks at all. If you are being recommended long-term hormone therapy, it is because the benefits of this form of treatment, which can be very great, far outweigh the risks described here.

A second class of side effect relates to the bones. It has been known for a long time that, after the menopause, women are more prone to developing osteoporosis, or thinning of the bones, sometimes leading to fractures. It seems that men on long-term hormone therapy might also be at increased risk of osteoporosis. A way of finding out whether you are at risk is to perform a special scan called a 'bone densitometry' scan. If this shows that your bones are becoming thin, or are at risk of becoming thin, it might be possible to treat you with a drug called a bisphosphonate, given either as a tablet or by injection, in order to reduce the risks. This has been shown to be very effective.

What you can do

- **Keep active** Hormone therapy tends to cause a loss of muscle mass, and a gain in weight. In view of this, and of the increased risks of diabetes, heart attacks, or strokes, regular exercise is a sensible thing to do if you can.

- **Try to keep your weight down** There is a tendency to put on weight with hormone therapy and avoiding this is difficult, but it is not impossible with careful attention to your diet.

- **Let your doctor know** if you develop symptoms such as chest pain, unusual thirst, and/or passage of unusually large amounts of urine. Ask whether you should have your bone mineral density measured.

7

Locally advanced disease

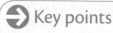 Key points

- Locally advanced disease is prostate cancer which has spread to the tissues immediately outside the prostate gland, but not elsewhere.

- It automatically defines the range of management and treatment options available

- The most common treatment is a combination of hormone therapy and radiotherapy, although some variations and alternatives are being tested.

What is locally advanced disease?

This somewhat alarming term is used to describe a prostate cancer which, although it has spread to the tissues immediately outside the prostate gland itself, has not given rise to detectable disease elsewhere, such as in lymph glands or bones. It is a more serious situation than disease confined to the prostate gland, for a number of reasons.

- It suggests that the type of cancer is likely to be one that would, untreated, cause problems to the patient (see Chapter 3). Hence it is more likely to need treatment, although this is not always the case (e.g. a slowly progressing tumour in an elderly patient with other significant illnesses might never cause problems within that patient's lifetime).

- It suggests that, if treated, surgery (a radical prostatectomy) would be unlikely to remove all the tumour, and other options, such as hormone therapy and radiotherapy (see below), are more likely to be appropriate.

◆ It is associated with a higher risk, at a later date, of developing prostate cancer in other parts of the body than is the case in patients with prostate cancer confined to the prostate gland.

None of the above suggests that the situation is hopeless—very far from it-although it is clearly more serious than in some other patients with prostate cancer. However, it does define the range of treatment and management options that might be appropriate.

Management

There are three main options for the management of locally advanced disease:

◆ watchful waiting

◆ radiotherapy

◆ hormone therapy.

The usual treatment in men who are fit is a combination of radiotherapy and hormone therapy. Recently, there has been more medical interest in surgery (radical prostatectomy) for some very carefully selected men with locally advanced disease, but this should only be done in a highly specialist centre and would not generally be recommended.

Hormone therapy for locally advanced disease

Hormone therapy is the mainstay of treatment for locally advanced and advanced prostate cancer. It is described more fully in Chapter 6, but some aspects of it will be reviewed again here. All forms of hormone therapy are designed to interfere with the male hormone, testosterone, which characteristically 'feeds' prostate cancer cells. Hormone therapy is sometimes referred to by other terms, such as androgen ablation therapy, androgen suppression therapy, or androgen deprivation therapy, but it all means the same thing.

There are four main ways of administering hormone therapy in locally advanced disease. They are all broadly as effective as each other, and the choice between them is made by a combination of the physician's preference and the patient's preference.

The oldest form of treatment is the bilateral orchidectomy (removal of both testicles, leaving the capsule of the testicle and the other contents of the scrotum intact).

An alternative to orchidectomy is a monthly injection (or, more recently, a three-monthly injection which is very long acting) of a drug which causes the level of testosterone in the blood to fall. This drug is called a LHRH agonist (luteinizing hormone-releasing agonist) or alternatively a gonadotrophin-releasing hormone (GnRH) agonist. These drugs are analogues of the hormone LHRH which is produced in the brain, and which stimulates the pituitary gland to produce the luteinizing hormone (LH). This, in turn, stimulates the testicles to produce testosterone. Because of the way in which these drugs act, they cause a transient but dramatic *rise* in testosterone levels for the first week or two after they are started, followed by a profound and dramatic fall in testosterone levels, equivalent to that seen after an orchidectomy. Because of this, LHRH agonists are usually combined with an anti-androgen (see below) for the first few weeks of treatment in order to protect against a so-called testosterone surge.

Recently, a new class of drug, called an LHRH antagonist, has been introduced. Unlike LHRH agonists, this drug does not cause a transient rise in testo-sterone levels and does not need to be given with oral anti-androgens at the start of therapy. These drugs are just coming into use for patients with advanced disease (see below), and trials are beginning in some men with locally advanced disease, or with localized disease where radiotherapy is being used.

It is also possible to interfere with the actions of testosterone using tablets called oral anti-androgens which, although they do not reduce the level of testosterone in the blood, block its actions on cells (normal and cancerous). It has been claimed that oral anti-androgens may have fewer side effects than other forms of hormone therapy, but not all specialists agree on this, and some feel that more data are needed to support this assertion. Because of anxieties that oral anti-androgens, by themselves, may not be as effective as other forms of hormone therapy (at least in men with advanced disease), this option is the least commonly used in men with locally advanced disease.

Irrespective of the mode of hormone therapy, the important 'bottom line' is that the response rates (i.e. the percentage of patients whose tumours will shrink significantly and/or whose blood PSA levels will fall significantly) are in excess of 85 per cent. Many of these responses are so-called complete responses, i.e. the tumour in and around the prostate gland shrinks to unde-tectable levels and the PSA level falls to within the normal range. They can also be long lasting in some patients, who continue hormone therapy long term, keeping the disease under control for some years. Unfortunately, as with hormone therapy for metastatic (advanced) disease, such responses cannot be guaranteed to last for the patient's lifetime and, indeed, would not do so for many otherwise fit men with locally advanced disease if hormone therapy was used alone. For this reason, hormone therapy is usually combined with radiotherapy in men who are fit enough to receive it. Also, importantly for the patient with symptoms from an enlarged prostate (such as frequency of urination, discomfort when urinating), hormone therapy will often result in an improvement in those symptoms (as discussed in Chapter 6).

Side effects

As with hormone therapy administered for other stages of the illness, patients may suffer from the same side effects, as discussed in more detail in Chapter 6. These include:

- impotence

- loss of libido (sexual desires)

- hot flushes

- some tendency to put on weight

- some reduction in the amount of facial and body hair.

Contrary to what is popularly believed, hormone therapy, even when done by removal of the testicles, does not cause the voice to become higher or breasts to grow, although some degree of breast enlargement may occur with some oral anti-androgens (see Chapter 6 for a fuller discussion of this). Additionally, it is now thought that hormone therapy given over a long period of time may result in an increase in other illnesses, notably diabetes and heart disease. Thinning of the bones (osteoporosis) is also recognized in some men, especially if their bones are showing a tendency to this when they begin hormone treatment. It is partly because of the side effects that, in patients with locally advanced disease, hormone therapy may be administered for a limited time, generally a few years, rather than indefinitely.

Impotence due to a loss of libido and an inability to achieve an erection, is one of the most significant problems associated with hormone therapy, and is discussed more fully in Chapter 12. It is worth noting that here that, after hormone therapy has stopped, normal sex function is only likely to recover when the body's testosterone levels have themselves recovered. This can take some months or even up to a year in the case of men who have had treatment with the three-monthly preparation of LHRH agonists. There are treatments which might help with erections, including tablets like Viagra or Cialis, and men who want to pursue these should be encouraged to start early, perhaps at the very onset of hormone therapy.

Radiotherapy for locally advanced disease

Radiotherapy (radiation therapy or X-ray therapy), as discussed in more detail in Chapter 4, consists of the use of high-energy X-rays (which are a form of radiation) which damage and kill cancer cells. They also damage and kill normal cells, but normal cells have a greater ability to repair radiation damage. Consequently, by carefully administering radiotherapy it is possible to completely destroy a cancerous tumour without also destroying the normal tissues which surround it.

Radiotherapy is often used in patients with locally advanced disease to treat the prostate gland plus the surrounding tissues, thus encompassing all of the tumour in a way that may not be possible with surgery. The technical aspects of radiotherapy, plus a fuller discussion of its side effects, are covered in Chapter 4, but are briefly reviewed again here.

Most commonly, in locally advanced disease, radiotherapy is administered as external beam therapy. This means that the patient lies on a couch, while an X-ray machine (usually a **linear accelerator**) directs a beam of high energy X-rays onto a carefully targeted area and in a carefully calculated dose. This is completely painless, and patients usually feel nothing while the machine is switched on. Patients are usually treated each day, from Monday to Friday, over 4–7 weeks (depending on the technique that is used). Each treatment takes around 15 minutes, most of which is spent setting up both patient and machine in the exact position required. Usually, daily treatment is given in three or four fractions with the machine in three or four different positions. Once the patient is in position, he usually maintains that position for each treatment while the machine is moved around him (see Chapter 4).

Side effects

The side effects of radiotherapy given in this context are the same as those discussed in Chapter 4 for patients receiving radiotherapy for disease confined to the prostate gland. Briefly, they can be divided into early (acute) side effects and delayed (late) side effects. Acute side effects are those which begin during the course of radiotherapy and may last for several weeks afterwards, while late side effects typically begin 6 months to 2 years after radiotherapy and can be permanent. All these side effects are discussed more fully in Chapter 5, and are only briefly reviewed here.

Acute side effects consist of an increase in frequency of urination, increased discomfort during urination, and a tendency to feel as if one needs to pass a large amount of urine, when only a small amount is actually passed. Patients often also experience increased frequency of passing bowel motions, sometimes with loose motions, diarrhoea, or even bleeding from the rectum. As with the urinary symptoms, patients may feel the need to pass a bowel motion urgently, only to find that they actually pass a small amount of motion, or even just mucus, slime, or blood. In addition, patients may feel generally tired and run down. Urinary side effects can be treated with a high fluid intake plus antibiotics where necessary, while bowel side effects can be treated with a low-fibre diet plus medication to combat diarrhoea.

Late side effects affect the bowel and/or bladder most commonly. If the bowel is affected, patients may experience looseness of motions and an increased frequency of passing motions (similar to those seen with acute side effects), which can vary in its extent from minor (e.g. bowels opened twice a day instead of once a day) to more severe (fortunately rare). Rectal bleeding may also occur with this, although it may be important for the doctor to exclude other causes. Similarly, late bladder side effects may manifest as similar symptoms to the acute effects, although they can be permanent in this context.

The other late side effect of importance is impotence, which may occur in upwards of 40 per cent of patients who were potent prior to radiotherapy. This is a consideration in patients whose hormone therapy has stopped, not all of whom will recover their potency when their testosterone levels recover.

Combined external beam radiotherapy plus brachytherapy

An extremely high dose of radiotherapy might be considered beneficial for some patients with locally advanced disease. This is usually achieved by a combination of external beam radiotherapy, as discussed above, plus brachytherapy. Usually, when brachytherapy is given in this situation, it is done in a slightly different manner to that used in men with localized disease (as discussed in Chapter 4), in that it uses **high-dose-rate brachytherapy**. This is done by inserting hollow needles into the prostate (similarly to the method for inserting radioactive seeds and under a general anaesthetic), which are used to introduce tubes which connect to a 'safe' containing small but highly active radioactive balls. When the patient has recovered from the anaesthetic, the radioactive balls pass down the hollow tubes and into the prostate, staying there for the prescribed period of time, and are then removed and returned to the 'safe'. Therefore this treatment is given as an inpatient procedure in one or more sessions, lasting between one and several days. After it is completed, the tubes are removed from the prostate and the patient is allowed to return home. This procedure, combined with radiotherapy, does seem to be a useful and well-tolerated treatment for some men and, as further evidence accumulates, it might become more commonplace in the future. It is not known at present whether giving a higher dose of radiotherapy using external beam techniques alone might be just as beneficial.

Watchful waiting

The evidence supporting the benefits of treatment for locally advanced prostate cancer is now well established. However, some men in this situation are elderly and may be unfit because of other medical conditions. In these circumstances, a recommendation may be made to treat with hormone therapy alone, reserving radiotherapy for use if the disease in the prostate gland is causing particular problems such as urinary symptoms which are not being controlled by the hormone therapy. Alternatively, in some men who are very unfit, and who have slowly growing but locally advanced disease, a policy of watchful waiting may be adopted. This is discussed further in Chapter 4.

TURP in locally advanced cancer of the prostate

In the same way that a benign prostate enlarges and causes blockage of the urethra, a malignant prostate can enlarge and cause the same type of symptoms. This can happen even when the disease otherwise appears to be under control. When this occurs, the surgeon may suggest a TURP. Some men will have had this procedure previously for benign enlargement of the prostate. Sometimes the operation requires to be performed a number of times and usually produces significant relief.

If a patient is not fit enough for a further TURP, insertion of a tube or catheter on a long-term basis may be suggested. This has the effect of allowing the bladder to drain and avoids an operation.

8

Advanced disease

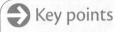 Key points

- Advanced disease is serious, and many patients in this situation have cancers that are not possible to cure.

- Hormone therapy results in regression of the cancer, often dramatically so, but it is unlikely to be permanent.

- If the disease comes back after hormone therapy, other options include different hormones, chemotherapy, bisphosphonates, and radiotherapy.

- In the near future, some new drugs might become available to combat this form of the disease.

What is 'advanced disease'?

Prostate cancers spread in several ways. They can spread via the lymphatic system (which helps to drain body fluids) to lymph glands in the pelvis, abdomen, chest, and neck (usually in that sequence). However, it is relatively less common to see lymphatic spread beyond the abdomen. Prostate cancers can also spread to other organs of the body via the bloodstream. Although many different organs can be involved, for some reason it is usually the bones that are particularly targeted by prostate cancers.

The term 'advanced disease' generally refers to cancers which have spread to other organs of the body, usually the bones. Patients whose prostate cancer has spread via the lymphatics to the abdomen or beyond are often treated in a similar manner to those with advanced disease, although some with lymph node metastases in the pelvis might be considered to have locally advanced disease.

Treatments for advanced or metastatic cancer

The mainstay of treatment for advanced disease is hormone therapy, which may also be referred to as androgen deprivation therapy or androgen suppression therapy. This has already been described in Chapers 6 and 7. However, patients with advanced disease are usually treated with indefinite long-term hormone therapy (although this may be changing as will be discussed below).

The chief limitation to hormone therapy as a treatment for advanced prostate cancer is that its benefits are nearly always temporary. That does not mean that it is not useful—quite the contrary—and it may control prostate cancer in some men for years. However, unless the man succumbs to an unrelated illness, his prostate cancer will eventually recur, and in that situation other treatments must be used.

Hormone therapy may be delivered by orchidectomy, LHRH agonists, LHRH antagonists, oral anti-androgens, or oestrogens. Orchidectomy and oestrogens are generally only given to men with advanced disease.

Orchidectomy

This means the surgical removal of the testicles. The testicles produce 90 per cent of the male sex hormones and the advantage of this operation means that hormone treatment is started at an early stage and also avoids injections or remembering to take drug treatments.

Of course, it is not reversible. It formerly enjoyed great popularity because it is a relatively cheap option, avoiding expensive drug bills over a period of time.

The disadvantages are obvious, in that a surgical operation and anaesthetic are required.

It appears to work as well as any of the drugs, and it is really a matter of personal preference as to which is undertaken. However, orchidectomy produces a more rapid fall in the level of testosterone (the male hormone) than is the case with some drugs. It will completely abolish sexual function.

The incision is made, usually through the scrotum, which is the bag that contains the testicles. Sometimes the surgeon will carry out a subcapsular orchidectomy, which leaves a small amount of tissue in the scrotum.

LHRH agonists

As discussed in Chapter 6, the usual form of hormone therapy is with an LHRH agonist. Recently, a new class of drug, called an LHRH antagonist, has been introduced and tested in randomized contolled trials. The effects of LHRH antagonists appear to be very similar overall, but anti-androgen tablets to prevent a 'flare' in the first few weeks (as described in Chapter 6) do not need to be given when an antagonist is used. Clinical trials are in progress to find out whether these drugs can be used in other situations, for example in locally advanced disease or even in early disease when radiotherapy is being used. Some of the first LHRH antagonists caused problems due to allergic reactions at the site of injection, but newer versions seem to have reduced, although not eliminated, this.

Intermittent hormone therapy

Conventionally, hormone therapy for men with advanced disease is given continuously, and for an indefinite time. However, clinical trials, started some years ago, attempted to determine whether it was detrimental to give hormone therapy intermittently. The usual way in which this is done is to give an initial course of treatment, say around 6–9 months, check that the PSA level has fallen adequately, and then stop hormone therapy and monitor the PSA. As and when the PSA begins to rise again, hormone therapy is reintroduced and the cycle is repeated. The main advantage is to allow men the prospect of a break from the side effects of hormone therapy, including (hopefully) a return of sexual function (although this may take some time). The chief concern, when this form of treatment was suggested, was that some men, who respond to hormone therapy the first time it is given, might fail to do so when it is given for a second time. Indeed, it appears that this is the case for a few men. However, overall, the results of clinical trials suggest that intermittent hormone therapy does not compromise survival. This form of therapy is slowly gaining in popularity, and although it is true that more clinical trial results are still awaited, it may be that this will become a much more widespread method of giving hormone therapy in the future.

Oestrogens

Oestrogens are female hormones, and it has been known since the 1940s that they can slow the growth of prostate cancer in men. The chief concerns are their side effects. In the early clinical trials, a form of oestrogen therapy called stilboestrol was used, but it caused an unacceptably high rate of cardiovascular problems, such as heart attacks and strokes, which were often fatal. It went out of fashion for that reason, but in the last few years it has been realized that it can be given at a much lower dose to that used in the original clinical trials, and with a much reduced (although not eliminated) risk of cardiovascular problems. Sometimes, in the lower dose, it is given with a small dose of soluble aspirin for added protection against these complications.

A clinical trial studying whether oestrogens can be given in a different form, as a patch which is put on the skin rather than by a tablet, is currently under way. There is evidence that, by using a patch, the cardiovascular side effects seen with oestrogen tablets such as stilboestrol might be reduced or even abolished.

Female hormones cause other side effects in men. Some enlargement of the male breast can occur, and may be painful. In some instances this might be prevented by giving a low dose of radiotherapy (often a single treatment) to the breasts. However, as with the other forms of hormone therapy, the voice does not change, and although beard growth may slow down, it does not usually stop altogether.

Disease worsening despite hormone therapy

This is a serious situation, but one in which an increasing number of treatments are becoming available. It used to be termed 'hormone-failed' or 'hormone-refractory' disease. It is now more commonly being referred to as 'castrate-refractory' prostate cancer (CRPC).

Despite these names, a **second-line hormone treatment** is often used, and may produce further responses. There is no 'best buy' in this situation, and the choice of drugs may be made from any of the options discussed in Chapter 6. However, following an orchidectomy or LHRH agonist therapy, the usual second-line hormone is an oral antiandrogen or stilboestrol (see above). Steroid therapy, using drugs such as prednisolone or dexamethasone, may work just like other forms of hormone therapy. Disappointingly, second-line responses are often neither as good nor as long as first-line responses.

The repertoire of other treatments in this situation used to be severely limited, but a number of options are now routinely discussed with patients:

Chemotherapy

Clinical trials of a type of chemotherapy using docetaxel have shown that this form of treatment is capable of prolonging the survival of men with CRPC. In addition, and importantly, it can improve quality of life and may reduce pain that is caused by prostate cancer. This has now become an accepted standard form of treatment for men in this situation, although it is generally used for men whose disease has spread to the bones and who are suffering from pain as a result. The duration of extra survival may be modest—around 3 months on average—but there is enormous variation from man to man, and some patients may survive for much longer while others derive no benefit.

Docetaxel is usually given as an outpatient therapy once every 3 weeks. It is delivered by injection, through a drip into a vein, and each treatment usually takes around an hour during which the patient is either sitting or lying down. Common side effects of this sort of chemotherapy include hair loss, reduction in the level of white blood cells (making a man more susceptible to infections), sore mouth, diarrhoea, skin and nail changes, soreness of the hands and feet, allergic reactions, a funny taste in the mouth, fluid retention, and tiredness. Docetaxel can also cause anaemia (because of a reduction in the number of red blood cells), and sometimes bruising or bleeding (because of a reduction in the number of blood platelets). Sickness and vomiting deserve some special mention and are discussed below. The list of side effects is indeed formidable, and this shows why it is important that chemotherapy is given by specialists in units that are equipped to deal with them. However, many patients will only experience a few of the side effects listed above, and it is very striking that, despite the long list of side effects, some patients who were getting symptoms from their prostate cancer actually feel better while on chemotherapy than they did before.

Sickness has long been recognized as a general side effect of many chemo-therapies and (together with hair loss) has been the most feared complication of chemotherapy. However, the last two decades have seen enormous progress in the development of drugs to combat nausea and vomiting. Today, the aim for every patient is that they should go through chemotherapy with *no* sickness at all! Do we achieve this? Realistically, no—there is often some degree of nausea, albeit usually mild, and in some patients we cannot prevent sickness. However, the experience of chemotherapy for the majority, while clearly unpleasant, is far from the nightmare that its reputation, or its past, would suggest. It is worth remembering that docetaxel chemotherapy is given as an outpatient, not an inpatient, procedure, and this must be testimony to how tolerable it actually is in practice.

When docetaxel is given, it is usually done in combination with steroid tablets (or injections). It is customary to give three to four cycles of chemotherapy before judging whether the disease has responded, and some men may go on to receive as many as 10 cycles of chemotherapy (30 weeks' duration)—again, a testimony to how tolerable this treatment often is in practice.

Close monitoring is important for patients on chemotherapy, and they will be advised about the 'warning signs' which, if they develop, should prompt a call to the treating hospital. In particular, a temperature, especially if the patient is feeling unwell, should prompt a call to the hospital, whatever the time of day or night, in case it is accompanied by a reduction in the number of white blood cells. Unfortunately, such a situation might necessitate a spell in hospital for a few days, and it is important that antibiotics are started promptly (maybe given by injection). It is worth buying a thermometer.

Bisphosphonates

These drugs predominantly target the bone, and their effect on prostate cancer is indirect. Like other types of cancer, prostate cancers, when in the bones, cause destruction of bone by recruiting the body's own bone cells. A type of cell, called the osteoclast, is responsible for digesting bone in normal situations, allowing new bone to be made (by cells called osteoblasts) in order to replace it. However, cancer cells may activate osteoclasts to digest bone excessively, and this seems to be as true of prostate cancers as other types of cancer despite the fact that, in prostate cancers, osteoblasts are also abnormally active.

Bisphosphonates inhibit the effects of osteoclasts, and by doing so they may reduce some of the problems caused by bone metastases (secondaries), including pain and even fracture of the bone due to excessive bone thinning and weakening. They are usually given, as an outpatient, by injection every 3–4 weeks, though some types may be given as a tablet. There are ongoing clinical trials to find out whether bisphosphonates are as effective as radiotherapy (see below) in relieving pain due to prostate cancer spread to bone.

Radiotherapy for prostate cancer pain

Patients with metastatic disease commonly have secondaries in the bones, which can be painful. **External beam radiotherapy**, given as a short course (e.g. five sessions) or even as a single treatment, is effective at relieving bone pain with minimal side effects. This is a different situation from the longer course of radiotherapy described in Chapter 4. An alternative is to use a radioactive drug, such as strontium or samarium, given by a single injection as an outpatient. This is as good as external beam radiotherapy in relieving pain, and in some patients may have the added advantage of preventing further pain in the short to medium term. Patients can return home after a strontium injection, though some minor precautions will need to be taken for a couple of weeks. In addition, a wide range of pain-killing drugs are now available, and can be given with the hope of major or complete pain relief in every patient. There is no reason for a patient with metastatic disease to suffer pain without having it adequately treated. Morphine is a superb pain killer, given for this reason and because of its flexibility in terms of dose, and *not because using morphine means that a patient is 'terminal'*. Addiction does not occur when morphine is given for cancer pain.

Other treatments for castrate-resistant prostate cancer

A number of other treatments have been, or are being, studied in clinical trials, and evidence is accumulating that they may be of benefit to patients with advanced CRPC. At the time of writing, they have not been introduced into clnical practice, although the next few years may well see the introduction of at least some of them. They include the following.

1. Immunotherapy: two drugs are currently under investigation, both of which boost the immune system and its response to prostate cancer, although in different ways. One is called sipuleucel-T, and it has been reported to improve the survival of men with CRPC, although further studies may be required. Another drug called ipilumumab is currently under study.

2. ZD4045 is a drug which targets a receptor called the endothelin receptor. Again, it has shown promise in clinical trials although, again, further studies may be needed.

3. A drug called abiraterone acetate deserves special mention, not so much because of its proven effectiveness, but because of the intense media frenzy that followed the reporting of the first (phase I) clinical trial in 2008. This led to a worldwide demand from patients and their partners, trying to get access to this drug (see Chapter 11), and is a good illustration of how a media story can engender false hope. Having said this, the drug is extremely promising for the stage of its development, the relevant phase III trials are under way, and it would not be surprising if these trials were to lead to its introduction. However, it cannot and should not be introduced before the trials are completed—there is no short cut.

This list is far from complete, but hopefully it serves to illustrate the enormous upsurge of interest in new treatments waiting in the wings for patients with prostate cancer. The future looks promising, but there is much still to do.

9

Alternative treatments

 Key points

+ Alternative treatments will often be regarded by physicians as a possible addition to standard treatment, not as a substitute.

+ Alternative treatments should always be discussed with your doctor first.

+ Alternative treatments include herbal therapies, visualization, and metabolic therapies.

The medical establishment can frequently appear as very authoritarian. When patients suggest alternative treatments, they are often greeted with a shrug, but rarely with any genuine interest on behalf of the physician. There are a number of physicians who are prepared to entertain alternative treatments, but almost all reputable physicians will suggest alternative treatments as an addition to standard treatment and not as a substitute.

It must be remembered that treatments that are orthodox today may have been considered alternative in the past. New treatments need to be scrutinized very carefully to assess whether they work and whether they are safe. Many alternative treatments are not regulated and are often not obtainable in many countries.

It is natural that patients should grasp at straws, and many of the practitioners in alternative medicine appear to be very articulate and caring. Almost all genuinely believe in the efficacy of their treatments, and occasionally they may appear as renegades, claiming that standard medicine and doctors do not take them seriously.

A sensible position will allow patients to pursue any alternative treatment that they may wish, as long is it is not harmful. It should be remembered that some of the alternative treatments are both unproven and occasionally dangerous.

Many of the alternative therapies would not be acceptable because they have not been proved to work and have not been subjected to the rigorous analysis of randomized controlled trials. However, conventional medicine does not know everything, and as long as the treatment is not harmful, then why shouldn't a patient try it, if he wishes? It is important to discuss this with the doctor first, however; the individual should beware the alternative practitioner who tries to persuade him not to do so.

Seeking some of these treatments arises out of a sense of guilt. Patients may feel that some defect in their behaviour, emotion, or religious faith may have brought a visitation of disease. Sir Ludwig Guttman asserted that happy people do not get cancer. He was laughed at initially, but it is now perceived that the nervous system has a much more profound effect on the body than was originally realized.

There has recently been considerable interest in a visualization technique to increase the effectiveness of the immune system. These techniques initially exploit the idea that a healthy mind will produce a healthy body. Counselling, hypnosis, and biofeedback can be used to promote greater emotional and spiritual well-being. It is occasionally claimed that these techniques change the course of an illness and induce remission.

There is no doubt that challenging life events, such as bereavement, lower the lymphocyte count, and so there may be a respectable scientific basis for pursuit of these types of treatment.

Non-drug drugs

In the course of development of new drugs, many plant extracts, fungi, etc. are analysed. Practitioners will claim that the use of one of their new agents will make a great difference to the cancer or to the patient's well-being.

Perhaps some of these new agents may prove to be of benefit, but one may care to ask why conventional drug companies have not bought them up, since they would make a fortune if they found a cure for prostate cancer.

In an experimental sense, a variety of newer agents are being tried. For example, shark cartilage, which is a natural food substance, is being studied carefully. However, it remains to be seen whether it will produce any real benefit for patients.

Immune therapies

A variety of remedies, usually herbal, have been claimed to boost the immune system. This should not be confused with more orthodox drugs, some of which are currently in conventional clinical trials, which are specifically designed to have a particular effect on the immune system. Some of the alternative immune system boosters are potentially toxic, however, and care must be taken with any physician who is not prepared to test his or her theories using standard controlled trials.

Herbal therapies

Various herbs have been used as potential treatments but, once again, the comments above about new agents hold true. One example from a few years ago that deserves special mention is PC-SPES, previously available in the USA. This has been investigated in clinical trials, and it appears that it has hormone-like effects and, indeed, probably works just like conventional hormone therapy. Whether it is actually 'better' than current conventional hormone therapy could only be tested in a randomized trial (see Chapter 11).

Metabolic therapies

This essentially applies a detoxification of the body, and anti-cancer diets, based on what are perceived as more natural foods (e.g. vitamins, minerals, and enzymes), which are alleged to cleanse the body. They are also alleged to repair damaged tissue and stimulate immune function. Of course, the body is quite capable of doing this on its own and there is no evidence that immune function and prostate cancer are diminished.

Once again, the patient who wishes to try these diets should feel free to do so if they are safe, and who knows?

As far as diet is concerned, there is no definite evidence that modifying diet after developing cancer makes any difference. Our own advice would be for the individual to take the advice of a physician in whom he has confidence. However, there are few circumstances when the general advice on a good diet—enough calories but not too many, less saturated fat, enough fresh fruit and vegetables—does not apply and it probably underpins the best dietary advice for all of us.

10

Chemo-prevention and vitamins

⮕ Key points

- There has been, and continues to be, research and developments into the possibilities of prevention of prostate cancer using tablets.

- Various other natural foodstuffs, drinks, vitamins, and compounds have been reported to reduce the chances of getting prostate cancer.

- Clinical trials using vitamins and natural foodstuffs have been disappointing so far, but research into these is ongoing.

There is an old adage that prevention is better than cure and many men, particularly those with a family history ask the very pertinent question: **'Can I do anything to prevent the disease developing?'**

There are a number of conditions diagnosed by biopsy of the prostate which are possibly pre-malignant lesions; in other words, they can turn into cancer. These are prostatic intra-epithelial neoplasia (PIN) and possibly proliferative inflammatory atrophy (PIA). True prevention may be difficult to achieve, since some of these treatments might have to take place in adolescence as data from post-mortems suggest that up to one-third of men in their thirties have early prostate cancer. There are effective agents which may work by slowing the growth and grade of progression of early prostate cancers.

Chemo prevention has used a class of drugs called 5-alpha-reductase inhibitors (men who do not have 5-alpha-reductase failed to develop even benign prostatic enlargement or prostate cancer). This led to the setting up of the Prostate Cancer Prevention Trial (PCPT). This showed that finasteride, one of the 5-alpha-reductase inhibitors, reduced the prevalence of prostate cancer compared with placebo.

Finasteride reduced prostate volume and improved urinary symptoms. The most unexpected finding was a small increase in the number of high-grade tumours (Gleason grade 7–10) detected at biopsy in the finasteride group, although some experts believe that this is an apparent and not a real increase because the drug changes the appearance of the prostate under the microscope.

More recently, a second trial, using a different drug called dutasteride, has been reported, once again suggesting a reduction in the number of prostate cancers developing, although this time without the apparent increase in high-grade tumours. However, it would be reasonable to conclude that these drugs, particularly dutasteride, might turn out to be useful in reducing cancers. If you are in a high-risk group, with a strong family history of the disease, you may wish to discuss this treatment with your doctor.

A new class of drug called selective estrogen receptor modulators (SERM) are showing some promise, but are still at the trial stage.

Antioxidants

Certain types of oxygen products in the body may interfere with DNA and may be carcinogenic. There are a number of compounds which act primarily as antioxidants, such as vitamin E, selenium, and lycopene.

Vitamin E

Vitamin E occurs naturally as a fat-soluble vitamin, but is added artificially to food stuffs such as margarine. At low dosage, the question of whether it works is debatable. What has become clear is that at high doses there is an increased rate of heart failure and all-cause mortality. Therefore vitamin E should be taken with caution, keeping within the recommended limits.

Selenium

Selenium is an essential trace element and its concentration depends on the concentration in the soil. Results from skin cancer trials observed a reduction in the incidence of prostate cancer, but this effect was most pronounced in those with an initial low serum selenium, many over 65 years of age. The SELECT study has been terminated, very disappointingly showing no evidence at all that selenium prevents prostate cancer. This highlights the importance of testing the use of vitamins and alternative medicines properly. Selenium was believed to increase the inhibitory effect of vitamin E.

Lycopene

Lycopene is found in tomatoes and also provides the red pigment in red fruits such as watermelon and grapefruit. Lycopene concentrations are higher in cooked tomatoes, but any effect is likely to be restricted to high intake. Tomatoes are certainly a palatable way of consuming lycopene and of course contribute to the 'five-a-day' fruit and vegetable intake, which is generally thought to reduce cancer, amongst other things.

Green tea

Prostate cancer is low in Asian countries and it is thought that polyphenols in green tea help with this. A variety of mechanisms have been proposed, but at present the evidence that green tea is helpful is probably no better than circumstantial. Nonetheless, it is a pleasant beverage and certainly unlikely to cause any harm.

Saw palmetto

This compound has been popular in the USA and seems to interfere with the action of testosterone. It has modest benefit in symptoms of benign disease. Its efficacy is slight and it has the added benefit that it appears to be harmless.

Vitamin D

The role of vitamin D in cancer prevention has been studied for many years. Populations living further from the equator have a higher overall cancer death rate. This suggests that increasing sun exposure, which increases vitamin D production could have preventative action in a variety of cancers. The evidence about the extent of sunshine exposure in vitamin D has been seen in as many as 13 different types of cancer. However, it is difficult to determine the role of Vitamin D in real life and it may be that it requires to be given as early as adolescence for it to have any effect at all. Indeed, a recent very large clinical trial was halted because of a lack of effect, but there may have been complex confounding factors behind this outcome. This is still an area of very active research, and some doctors will routinely measure the levels of vitamin D in a patient's blood, although the evidence that this is beneficial is not conclusive.

Non steroidal anti-inflammatory drugs

Recent studies of the effects of aspirin in prostate cancer risk found a very modest reduction in those taking this drug. However, long-term regular use appears to be important. Other non-steroidal anti-inflammatory drugs have been associated with well-publicized problems and should only be taken on medical advice.

Statins

This is a fairly new field and there is a small amount of evidence that statins decrease cancer risk because of their anti-inflammatory effect. The benefit is probably not sufficient to warrant taking a statin, unless there are other reasons to do so, but those who are already on statins may take comfort from the fact that there is a possibility that this is also reducing cancer risk!

Fish oils

Despite early promise, the hope that fish oils would reduce prostate cancer has not been realized. Investigation of fatty acids appears to be complicated by the realization that it is the ratio of saturated to unsaturated fats, rather than the absolute levels, which may influence risk.

Other compounds

Pomegranate juice is a strong antioxidant which is receiving attention, and further trials are necessary to see what the effects are. Certainly if you like pomegranate juice, it would appear at least to do you no harm!

11

Clinical trials

➡ Key points

◆ Clinical trials have been essential in the development of cancer treatments. There is evidence that patients in clinical trials generally do better than patients not in a trial.

◆ All clinical trials have practical advantages and disadvantages, and you should discuss these with your specialist team.

◆ Cancer clinical trials are classified in three phases: phase I, phase II, or phase III studies.

◆ A clinical trial can only be undertaken if the doctor and the patient feel comfortable with it—it's OK to say 'no'!

What is a 'clinical trial'? Its very name conjures up images—Perhaps a courtroom? Trials and tribulations? Using patients as 'guinea pigs'? However, clinical trials have played a vital role in the development of cancer treatments. Without them, we would lack many of the important cancer treatments that are now available. It is well known that the use of clinical trials to test and develop new cancer treatments is widely supported by the majority of the population, and yet relatively few people are prepared to enter a clinical trial themselves—perhaps rightly? Whatever the reasons, or the rights and wrongs, it is a fact that, in the UK, only some 10 per cent of cancer patients are ever treated within the context of a clinical trial, and the figure is lower than this for prostate cancer patients in some parts of the UK. Before discussing the advantages and disadvantages of clinical trials, we first need to discuss what a clinical trial is, and how it is designed.

Design and conduct of clinical trials of cancer treatment

Conventionally, cancer treatments are evaluated in trials which are classified as phase I, II, or III studies. Phase I and II studies apply particularly to new drugs that are being introduced, and phase III studies apply to a range of treatment options including radiotherapy, drug therapy, and hormone therapy. Phase III studies involve the comparison of two or more treatment strategies. In prostate cancer, there have, historically, been relatively few phase I and II studies compared with other cancer types, but this situation is gradually changing as new treatments are being developed.

Phase I studies

In a phase I study, a new drug is tested in patients with a range of cancers, whose illness is active and who have already received all conventional anti-cancer treatments. More rarely, such a study may be performed in healthy volunteers. Its aim is to discover the correct dose of the new drug, and to obtain an understanding of its side effects and characteristics when used in humans. Usually this means starting the drug at a very low dose—defined by laboratory studies—and gradually increasing the dose until side effects prevent any further increase (the so-called 'dose-limiting toxicity' has been defined). Although it is hoped that a new drug in a phase I study will demonstrate anti-cancer activity—and such activity is always closely looked for and monitored—it is not in itself the primary goal, which is to define the correct dose and means of administration of the drug. More detailed study of anti-cancer activity is the remit of the phase II study.

Phase II studies

Phase II studies depend on the outcome of a phase I study, in that the starting point is that the best dose schedule is already worked out. Patients with a particular type of cancer (e.g. prostate cancer), whose illness is active and who have already received all available conventional anti-cancer treatments, are then treated with the new agent and are closely monitored for signs of anti-cancer activity. It is particularly at this stage of investigation that the promise of new agents might first become evident. If such promise is demonstrated, the drug will proceed to phase III studies. If not, as unfortunately is the case in the majority of new agents, it is unlikely to be developed further for that particular cancer type.

Phase III studies—the randomized controlled trial (RCT)

Phase III studies involve a formal comparison of two or more treatment strategies using single drugs, combinations of drugs, or combinations of treatment types (e.g. radiotherapy, hormone therapy). An important feature of these studies is that the selection of treatment is up to neither the patient nor the doctor, but is decided at random by an outside source (e.g. a computer in a trials office). This is why such studies are referred to as 'randomized trials', and it is this aspect of them which is most perplexing to patients—and to doctors.

Why 'randomize'?

The reason for randomization is to eliminate bias. Everybody is biased—doctors, patients, nurses—to a greater or lesser extent. However, it might be argued that, as long as the patients are well matched, they should be allowed to choose a treatment option freely in a trial, as should their doctors. Let us examine the reasons why this is not the case.

Imagine a new treatment—let us call it ABC12345—which is to be given alongside hormone therapy for prostate cancer. This treatment has been designed by a doctor who is conducting a trial comparing the survival rates of patients treated with either hormone therapy alone or hormone therapy plus ABC12345, and he decides not to use randomization.

The first patient, Mr Smith, comes to the outpatient clinic. He is aged 50, a keen athlete, and does not smoke. He has had a prostate cancer diagnosed, which did not look aggressive under the microscope, and his PSA level is only slightly raised. The doctor decides that he is an ideal candidate for ABC12345 therapy. The second patient, Mr Jones, comes to the clinic. Unlike Mr Smith, he is 78, is a heavy smoker, and weighs 18 stone. He had a large aggressive-looking cancer diagnosed and has a very high PSA level. The doctor decides that he should not be treated with ABC12345, but should receive hormone therapy alone.

Five years later, the doctor observes that Mr Smith is alive and well but, sadly, Mr Jones died only 2 months after his visit to outpatients. He concludes that ABC12345 is an effective treatment for prostate cancer, but is he right? Might Mr Jones's demise not be related to his general fitness, or to his more aggressive disease, rather than being related to the fact that he did not receive ABC12345? Mr Smith and Mr Jones were not comparable—there was a bias on the part of of the doctor in selecting the fittest patient for his new therapy.

Patients can also be biased. If they had been given the choice of treatment, Mr Smith might have opted for ABC12345, as an extra 'insurance' against his cancer returning, whereas Mr Jones might have decided against it because he already had many hospital appointments, was already taking 10 types of tablets every day, and did not want to take any more or have any extra hospital visits.

These are biases which, it could be argued, we can broadly identify, and perhaps do something about. The problem is that for every source of bias that is obvious, there tend to be others that are not obvious, and which may only become apparent many years later. These factors may be biological, for example characteristics of an illness associated with a particular activity or background that we do not know about. They may be similar to those discussed, but less obvious. For all these reasons, it is recognized that randomization is the best defence against sources of bias, known or unknown, interfering with the correct interpretation of a phase III study, and the randomized trial is regarded as the international gold standard by which a new treatment strategy is judged.

The benefits of clinical trials

Immediate benefits (to the trial participants)

As a broad generalization, patients benefit from being treated within the context of clinical trials, almost irrespective of what the particular trial is about. This has been shown in a number of studies which have looked at the quality of care and the survival of patients while treated within the context of a randomized trial. Not only is the quality of care generally better for patients when treated as part of clinical trial, but they tend to survive for a longer period of time than do comparable patients not treated in the context of a trial. There are probably many reasons for this, among them being that hospitals which participate in clinical trials do, by and large, have a very high standard of clinical practice. In addition, patients in a clinical trial are generally monitored more closely, and a have a closer relationship with clinical staff, than patients who are being treated 'routinely' outside a trial setting.

It is impossible to guarantee that every patient will benefit in this manner, but the very least that can be said is that, by its very nature, the treatment package that a patient would receive within a clinical trial would be the 'best' available, since no clinical trial would be permitted by the professional, research, or lay ethical bodies if this were not the case.

Longer-term benefits (to mankind)

It goes without saying that no clinical trial would be permitted if it were not attempting to answer some question that was of genuine and substantial importance. Previous questions which have been answered by randomized clinical trials include the treatment of breast cancer by a 'lumpectomy' (removal of a breast lump alone) rather than by a full mastectomy, the use of tamoxifen and chemotherapy to prolong the survival of women with breast cancer following their surgery, the use of newer forms of radiotherapy for the treatment of lung cancer (or, as we have seen, for high-dose conformal radiotherapy for prostate cancer), or the use of chemotherapy for other types of cancer, including cancer of the colon. Many of these are now regarded as 'standard', yet none of them would currently be possible, had previous generations of patients not consented to take part in the randomized trials that tested them. There is always a certain element of altruism in taking part in clinical research. Indeed, many consent forms contain the phrase 'I understand that this trial may not be of benefit to me, but may be of benefit to other patients in the future'.

In the case of prostate cancer, there are more unanswered questions than there are in many other types of cancer. In almost no other area of common cancer is there such a great need for research, using clinical trials, to test and compare treatments in order to answer some of these questions. Despite this, it has proved to be harder to conduct clinical trials in prostate cancer than in many other types of cancer. This is changing, and recently a number of clinical trials have been analysed, which prove (among other things) that higher radiotherapy doses are better than lower doses at treating the prostate itself, that chemotherapy with docetaxel prolongs the lives of men with advanced prostate cancer (albeit only modestly), and, most recently, that PSA screening might prevent some men from dying of prostate cancer, but at the price of exposing many more men to unneccesary treatment with its attendant risks. Nonetheless, there are some very good reasons why it is difficult to conduct randomized trials in prostate cancer. Some of the treatments that need to be tested are very different in their nature and in their implications to the patient. For example, the comparison of surgery, radiotherapy, and surveillance is universally regarded as being one of the most important of the unanswered questions about the treatment of 'early' prostate cancer. For some patients, these treatment options are so different that it is difficult or impossible to accept the idea of being allocated one of them by a random process. Despite this, the team in the UK conducting a clinical trial called ProtecT has now succeeded in recruiting around 1600 men to just such a trial, although the results will not be available for some years to come.

The next few years will tell us whether it is possible to conduct randomized trials of many of the aspects of prostate cancer treatment. If not, time may be running out, and both doctors and patients might have to accept that there are certain questions that society has determined are best left unanswered. The philosophical implications of such a conclusion are of an enormity that goes far beyond the remit of this book.

The drawbacks of clinical trials

The hazards to participants

Just as no cancer treatment can be considered to be entirely without risk, no clinical trial can be considered to be entirely without risk. Many of the risks will consist of the standard side effects and complications of cancer treatments, although if a new treatment is also be considered, it may have unrecognized problems that will only appear during the course of a clinical trial. The essential point is that patients are made fully aware of the hazards of any clinical trial before they agree to participate. This is demanded by professional and research bodies, generally agreed by defining ethical and moral principles that were enshrined in the Helsinki Declaration.

If the risks cannot be entirely eliminated, then it is axiomatic that they must be acceptable. As a guiding principle, a doctor should not enter a patient into a clinical trial he would not himself be prepared to enter, or have a member of his family entered into. Clinical trials can only be undertaken if the doctor and the patient are comfortable with the design and the immediate implications of the actual trial.

The restrictions on doctors

In order to protect both doctors and patients, a number of restrictions are placed on the launching and conduct of a clinical trial. Before trials can be considered, the scientific background has to be accepted by a respected scientific body, such as the UK Medical Research Council, Cancer Research UK, or the scientific committee of another medical charity. In addition, many hospitals have their own scientific committee which will scrutinize proposed new clinical trials, and these will include some of the very important studies of new drugs which have been designed by the pharmaceutical industry. The process of scientific approval can be very long, and may involve the examination of the proposed trial by a succession of different committees in that organization. This applies particularly to the major cancer charities and the Medical Research Council. In some instances, this can take several years.

Having made the scientific case for undertaking a clinical trial, and having persuaded the professional bodies that it is morally and ethically right to do so, a trial has to be passed by a regional ethical committee made up of both healthcare professionals and lay members. This body will also expect to be kept informed about progress of the trial and, in due course, trial results. In many instances, an independent data monitoring committee of experts will be appointed, which reviews the conduct of the trial and provides an independent assessment as to whether the progress of the trial justifies its continuation. For example, if in a comparison of treatments, one treatment appears to be showing superior results to another, the data monitoring committee may order the cessation of trial on ethical grounds.

It's OK to say 'no'!

Having described the importance of clinical trials, and having recognized the safeguards which are built into them to protect both patients and doctors, it is worth repeating the statement that a clinical trial can only be undertaken if the doctor and the patient feel comfortable with it. This will not always be the case—every patient is different, and every individual will have his or her own bank of experience, concepts, and beliefs. Some patients will not wish to take part in clinical trials offered, and it is entirely proper that they should feel free not to do so. It is almost more important than all the safeguards, that patients who decline the offer of entering a clinical trial should feel that the care that they will receive will be the best available, and that they can refuse (or even change their mind at a later date, having already entered a trial) without any worry as to the implications that this may have. A hospital taking part in a clinical trial is likely to have a very high standard of practice, and no doctor will take it as a personal insult if the patient does not want to take part in clinical research. Consent to take part in a clinical trial must be freely given, and must be an informed choice.

The media: publicity and 'hype'

Cancer research is 'big business'. Charities depend on the steady flow of income to maintain their research base, and cancer stories are always popular items for the media. On the basis that, in order to sell newspapers, there has to be a good story, it is unfortunately the case that a clinical study that suggests that a new treatment may be beneficial is more likely to find its way into the media than a study that suggests no particular benefit. Equally, there is a tendency on the part of the media to 'hype' a new cancer treatment, even if the research suggesting its possibilities is at a very early stage. The road to a new cancer treatment is long and arduous, and many treatments which look promising in the early stages of research turn out to be without benefit, or to offer no particular advantages over and above those of existing treatments.

Some cancer stories are genuinely 'big' stories. However, for the majority, there is a danger that the story will raise false hopes, and patients who are distressed, and therefore very vulnerable, will often want to explore anything new that is reported the media. The doctor's responsibility is to provide that patient with an honest appraisal of the scientific evidence relating to a particular story, and if a particular new treatment is either inappropriate or unavailable, then he must be told this honestly and sympathetically.

Parting shot—'more' is not always 'better'!

One common clinical trial design is one in which the new treatment is added to an existing one, and this sort of design confers particular difficulties for patients. For example, an ongoing clinical trial in prostate cancer is investigating whether the addition of radiotherapy is beneficial for certain patients who are being treated with hormone therapy.

Why do this as a randomized clinical trial? Surely, it might be reasonably argued, if there is any suspicion that 'more' treatment might be better, it would be reasonable simply to add that treatment. After all, the results of many treatments for cancer are unsatisfactory, and anything that might make them better is fully justified. Indeed, some people say that it is irresponsible not to simply add whichever extra treatments are available, and that a failure to do so is merely another example of economic stringency.

This seemingly sensible argument rests on one assumption—additional treatment is only likely to be beneficial, and will not be harmful. Unfortunately, we already know that this is not the case. The best example of this has come from a detailed analysis of all studies examining the addition of radiotherapy to surgery for patients with lung cancer. This might be expected to be a situation where extra treatment could only benefit patients, but, rather surprisingly, the reverse was the case. The survival of patients who were treated with a combination of surgery and radiotherapy was actually worse than the survival of patients treated with surgery alone. Modern cancer treatments are powerful, and we cannot simply add the treatments without testing such a combination in a formal way.

12

Prostate cancer and sex

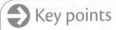 Key points

- Sex is part of healthy living for all of us.

- An active sex life may be possible after diagnosis with prostate cancer.

- A variety of drugs available to treat erectile dysfunction (ED).

- Drugs bought over the Internet may not come from reputable sources and may not work properly or at all.

- Penile inserts or prostheses are possible, but are often used as a last resort.

Sex is part of healthy living for all of us. The sexual urge decreases in most men with time. Nonetheless, it is well known that men can father children well into their eighties. A woman's interest in sex may decrease after the menopause, but this is not necessarily so. Most men who have prostate cancer are not in the first flush of youth, and for some couples sexual activity may have virtually stopped in any case. For some men, even elderly men, the inability to have intercourse can be devastating. For others, it may not matter. Neither instance is 'right' or 'wrong'.

Impotence

Impotence can be both mental or physical. Impotence is defined as the inability to achieve and maintain a firm enough erection to permit penetration in intercourse.

Impotence can occur in any age group. It is probably true to say that most men have a period of impotence at some stage in their life. This can be caused by depression, bereavement, etc. As men get older, frequency of intercourse and penile rigidity gradually reduce. In some men, the male sexual hormone may decrease significantly with age.

Being given the diagnosis of cancer is, of course, unlikely to improve your sex life and it can take a number of months for patients to adjust to this knowledge. One reaction is that the patient thinks that cancer has been visited upon him for some reason, perhaps due to previous sexual encounters or perceived bad conduct at some stage. A perception of being 'unclean' may develop and it is important that the spouse understands what may appear to be rejection. Another anxiety that male patients have is that they may pass on their disease in some way to their wives. This is just not possible and is not a reason to abstain from intercourse. Patients should also be reassured that sexual intercourse will not accelerate or alter the disease. Many of the treatments of prostate cancer will produce either complete or partial impotence, and the consultant should have discussed this with each patient.

Although these questions can be embarrassing, one should not feel embarrassed about asking the urologist. The urologist deals with many men for a wide variety of sexual problems and he or she may merely assume that an individual who does not enquire is not interested in asking. The condition is now known as ED or erectile dysfunction

Treatments

Phospho-diesterase type 5 inhibitors

This is an important group of pills for ED.

Viagra (sildenafil) and Revatio

Of the various treatments available for impotence, one of the best known is Viagra (sildenafil). Two brands are now available. This probably does not work quite so well in patients with prostate cancer, but it is certainly worth trying. The usual starting dose is 50 mg, as a tablet, taken about an hour before sexual activity. This may be reduced to 25 mg in elderly men, and the largest single dose is 100 mg, which is available as a separate tablet. Erections may not occur spontaneously and genital manipulation may be required. It is recommended that the drug is not repeated for 24 hours. Sildenafil is contraindicated in men on glyceryl trinitrate (GTN) tablets or in patients with a recent history of stroke or heart attack. It should also be avoided in patients with low blood pressure and, rarely, in patients with disorders of the retina of the eye. This drug is not available on the NHS for all patients with erectile dysfunction, but is available for patients who have had treatment for prostate cancer, particularly those who have had radical prostatectomy or other forms of pelvic surgery. The side effects include headache, flushing of the face, dizziness, and, in some people, disturbance of blue–green colour perception. Nasal congestion can also occur. It is important that urgent medical attention is sought if an erection lasts for more than 4 hours.

Tadalafil (Cialis) 10–20 mg

The effect of this medication may last more than 24 hours, but erection does not (or should not) persist for this length of time. The dosage is restricted to once daily and many patients like the more prolonged effect.

Vardenafil (Levitra) 10–20mg

This is an alternative to sildenafil.

Alprostadil (MUSE)

The dosage of the pellet, which is placed in the urethra at the opening of the penis, is 250 µg and it is recommended that this be used no more than twice in a 24-hour period. Some people experience stinging when the drug is inserted.

Injections into the penis

Alprostadil is prostaglandin E_1. It is given by self-administered injection. Some preparations come as a powder, which has to be made up with fluid, which is also supplied. The injection is into the shaft of the penis. The initial dose is 5 µg, which may be increased up to 20 µg, with a maximum of 40 µg. It is recommended that this injection is used only once in one day and no more than two or three times in any one week. Special training must be given to patients before they use it.

Vacuum pumps

Vacuum devices have their place for certain individuals. The penis is placed in a vacuum chamber (do not under any circumstances use a vacuum cleaner) and a pump is used to create a vacuum, allowing blood to be drawn into the penis. A constriction ring is slipped on to the base of the penis to trap the blood in the penis, allowing intercourse. It is important to obtain a system that is reliable. Many inferior brands leak.

Surgical implants

Very occasionally, patients may wish to explore the use of a penile implant. This can be either rigid or inflatable. The operation destroys the erectile tissue, thus making any future treatment redundant. It is our opinion that these devices may have a place, but it should be remembered that the enjoyment which is given is almost exclusively to the female and the insertion of these devices stops any attempt at further drug treatment.

13

Questions and answers

Q *What are the early symptoms of prostate cancer?*

A Early prostate cancer does not usually have symptoms.

Enlargement of the prostate can cause difficulty passing water, blood in the water, and a reduction in urinary stream. This is usually caused by what is called benign enlargement of the prostate (also called benign prostatic hyperplasia or BPH).

Q *What is the difference between a tumour and cancer?*

A A tumour involves enlargement of any group of cells within the body. Tumours can be benign or malignant. Benign tumours may cause problems locally by enlargement, such as reduction of urinary stream. However, they are not malignant. Cancers have two properties which cause them to be malignant—they can invade locally and they can spread to distant sites.

Q *How do tumours kill people?*

A Tumours can kill people by various mechanisms. First, they can run away with all the essential foodstuffs that the body requires, and while the body is starving, the tumour is growing at the expense of its host. Secondly, growing tumours cause local damage and obstruction. For example, tumours growing within the central nervous system can cause problems with the circuitry of the nervous system, and secondary tumours growing in the liver can press on the bile ducts and cause jaundice. Thirdly, tumours can produce substances which cause the rest of the body to malfunction.

Q *Can benign tumours become malignant?*

A There is very little, if any, evidence to suggest that benign enlargement of the prostate turns into malignancy. Benign enlargement of the prostate is extremely common and most men will have some degree of this within their lives.

Q *Why is cancer so common?*

A The question really should be why, with all the numbers of dividing cells within the body, is cancer not more common? It tends to get more common as we get older and this is mainly due to DNA damage and also reaction to agents, such as viruses, that subvert the normal pattern of cell replacement.

Q *How quickly does the cancer grow?*

A Different cancers grow at different rates. Some men's prostates may harbour it for very many years before it becomes clinically evident. Some unfortunate men have very aggressive forms of cancer, and these can grow at a great rate and cause death within a very short space of time.

Q *Can I catch cancer from someone?*

A Prostate cancer is not transmitted either from male to female or male to male.

Q *Does the body have natural defences against cancer?*

A The body has a whole variety of defences against abnormal cell growth. The DNA, which is the construction plan for each cell, is kept within the nucleus of each cell. There are highly adapted packaging proteins for DNA called histones, which package the DNA in clumps. The DNA itself has two chains, both of which are complementary, which means that if one strand is damaged, the opposite strand can still provide a template for the DNA to be replaced without change.

Various enzymes control the defence of the DNA. If a cell becomes damaged, there is an actual mechanism to cause it to die, and this is called apoptosis. If a cell becomes too much of a renegade, it can develop different cell coatings. The immune system constantly patrols the cells of the body and in many circumstances might pick up abnormal cells and kill them. It does this to control both cancer and any bacteria which enter the system.

Q *Can I reduce the risk of prostate cancer?*

A There is no foolproof way of reducing the risk. Although there is a slight association with smoking, it could not be said that smoking is strongly associated with prostate cancer. However, here are sufficient reasons to give up smoking without looking at prostate cancer risk. A normal healthy diet should contain enough vitamins and antioxidants to prevent cancer.

If you are eating a normal healthy balanced diet, with enough fruit and vegetables (e.g. five items of fruit and vegetables per day), it should not be necessary to top up the level of naturally occurring vitamins. Small amounts of proprietary vitamins will not do any harm, but there are instances where particular vitamins, such as vitamin A, can in fact be harmful. Too much vitamin C predisposes you to develop stones in your urinary tract. For men at very high risk of prostate cancer, new evidence for drugs such as dutasteride should be discussed with the doctor.

Q *Is there a connection between cancer and emotional states?*

A Sir Ludwig Guttman used to state that happy people do not get cancer. It was originally thought that he was making an unsupportable statement, despite his evidence in dealing with spinal injuries, and his comments were laughed at.

Nowadays we are not so sure. There is unquestionably a link between the immune system and positive attitudes. It can certainly be said that none of the emotional treatments do any harm and many people find it at worst a comfort in their time of trial.

In certain illnesses, visualization of the tumour has been thought to be helpful, and there is a whole new science of psychobiology where patients are given support to deal with their illness.

Q *My father died of prostate cancer at age 55. Do I have an increased chance of developing the disease?*

A Current evidence suggests a modest degree of increased risk with one close relative affected, increasing if more than one are affected. It is worthwhile discussing this further with the specialist, although it is unknown whether monitoring (or 'screening') is effective. Less commonly, men from families who carry a gene mutation (e.g. in the breast cancer genes BRCA1 or BRCA2) may be found, and they may have an increased risk of prostate cancer. Sometimes a discussion with specialists in medical genetics might be helpful if you have a strong family history of breast cancer or prostate cancer.

Q *If there is an increased chance, should I be on a screening programme?*

A The British Government has now decided that any patient wishing to have his PSA tested can have this done. It is important that this test is understood fully (see Chapters 3 and 5).

It is worth reflecting that patients are very keen to have a negative PSA test, but the question to ask yourself is: 'In the event that I have a positive test, would I wish to go on to a transrectal ultrasound and biopsy, given that if that shows prostate cancer, the treatment options are not clearly defined?'

Q *What are the options if screening indicates a rising PSA level?*

A The options are:

- to do nothing and disregard it

- to have the PSA monitored

- to ask for a urological/oncological opinion

- through a urologist, ask for a transrectal ultrasound and biopsy, if it is felt appropriate.

Q *What are the chances that there is spread of this disease?*

A It rather depends on how advanced the disease is when it has been discovered. In the past almost 50 per cent of people had advanced disease, but now patients who are having their PSA tested are being identified at a much earlier stage, and the number of men presenting in this way in the UK is around 20 per cent. In the USA, very few men have advanced disease when they are first diagnosed.

Q *Can the specialist tell if my cancer will spread?*

A Unfortunately, it is not possible to tell with any certainty. Gleason scores that are higher indicate more likelihood of spread than those that are lower, but there is no one feature that tells us which is going to be a 'tiger' and which is going to be a 'pussycat'.

Q *What is my life expectancy?*

A This rather depends on how advanced your tumour is. It is comforting to note that many patients who were followed up in Scandinavia, who had in fact received no treatment, survived in excess of 10 years. Perhaps they were lucky, but nonetheless a diagnosis of prostate cancer does not necessarily indicate that it will be the cause of death.

Q *Can my cancer be cured (I am more interested in survival than my sex life)?*

A As a rough estimate, all patients who have PSAs less than 10, and have early prostate cancer with a Gleason sum score less than 7, have a better than 50 per cent chance of being alive and well 10 years later. This per-centage is probably also the case for patients having radical radiotherapy or surgery.

Q *If it is not curable, can it be controlled?*

A Hormonal treatment is capable of keeping early disease at bay for many years. Occasionally, radical treatment can be combined with hormonal treatment and once again this can control the disease for many years.

Q *Do I actually need treatment (cancer confined to prostate gland)?*

A This is something that you should discuss in detail with your urologist or oncologist. No reputable surgeon or oncologist would mind if you asked for a second opinion. In the USA, it is not uncommon for patients to have two, three, or even four opinions before opting for treatment. The Internet can be a great source of information, but remember that the Internet is not quality controlled and that some of the information is not without bias.

Q *Why do doctors disagree about what is best (three doctors, three treatments)?*

A The real reason for this is that there have been few randomized controlled trials in early prostate cancer. All the evidence that is used is circumstan-tial. If your doctor is being honest with you, he will find it fairly perplexing and even asking the question 'What would you have done yourself doctor?' would not necessarily meet with a realistic answer. Your doctor has almost certainly not been diagnosed with prostate cancer himself and none of us can really know what this is like until we have been diagnosed.

Q *Active monitoring may not be 'active' enough! What can I do for myself (diet, sex)?*

A It is probably fair to say that there is very little you can do, other than lead as normal a life as you can and try to forget about your diagnosis as much as possible. Life is for enjoying—it is important that you continue with all your normal activities, including sexual intercourse, if you are able. There is no evidence that altering diet improves survival and you should eat what you feel is best for *you*.

Q *What are the disadvantages of active monitoring?*

A The main argument here is that the genie can escape from the bottle; in other words, cancer cells, untreated, can spread from the prostate gland. With careful watchful waiting and surveillance of PSA, there is no evi-dence that your chances of survival are impaired.

Q *I have had treatment for prostate cancer. How often should I be seen by my specialist?*

A This is best determined in consultation with your urologist, oncologist, or GP. Three- to six-monthly seems appropriate in most cases.

Q *What are the treatment options if active monitoring culminates in the progression of prostate cancer?*

A Assuming that the cancer has not become more advanced, the options are the same as early treatment, mainly radical prostatectomy, radical radio-therapy, or brachytherapy.

Q *If I wait, will it be more difficult to treat in the future and how fast will it spread?*

A Assuming that you have been under proper surveillance, it is unlikely that the disease will advance to such a state that it becomes untreatable. It is important that you ensure that you and your medical adviser are speaking about the same things. Unfortunately it is unlikely that we can tell with any accuracy how fast the cancer will spread (the pussycat and tiger story).

Q *If I have treatment, should this be with surgery or radiotherapy?*

A This is a matter for discussion and debate. There are advantages and dis-advantages with both forms of treatment. Unfortunately, there is no firm evidence that one is 'better' than the other, provided that treatment is of the highest quality. The choice is often determined by the balance of the possible side effects (see Chapter 4).

Q *What are the possible adverse side effects of radical prostatectomy?*

A As has been discussed earlier, these are incontinence, impotence, blood loss, and death.

Q *Who would you choose to do your operation?*

A It makes sense to choose a surgeon who is experienced and can tell you what his or her particular incontinence and impotence rates are.

Q *What are the early (temporary) side effects of radiotherapy?*

A These include disturbance of bladder function, diarrhoea, and mucus pro-duction from the rectum.

Q *What are the late (permanent) side effects of radiotherapy?*

A These are similar to the temporary effects, but they are permanent.

Q *What are the roles of hormone therapy?*

A Hormone therapy is an excellent way of reducing the effect of the male sex hormone, testosterone, on all forms of prostate tissue, including prostate cancer. In most cases, this does not result in a cure, but rather defers and holds off the disease, usually for about 2 years but sometimes much longer. Many thousands of patients have been entered into studies to try and determine this. The idea is that maximum androgen blockade not only interferes with testicular hormones, but also deals with testosterone produced by the adrenal gland. However, studies suggest that the benefits of maximum androgen blockade are small or marginal, and it is not routinely used in the UK.

Q *How can the side effects of treatment be minimized?*

A One side effect that can be quite tedious is hot flushes (called this in the UK, but called hot flashes in the USA). These are usually abolished by using a small daily dosage (50 mg) of cyproterone acetate (Cyprostat, Androcur). Bicalutamide (Casodex) has a major side effect, in that it causes enlargement of the male breasts which can be painful. In some cases, oncologists may offer you a small dose of radiotherapy to each breast prior to starting this.

Q *What about my sex life?*

A Impotence is a problem with almost all the treatments. It is less of a problem with bicalutamide and flutamide than with other forms of hormone therapy, and it may be lower with brachytherapy than with surgery or radiotherapy. Your doctor should discuss the importance of sexual function with you, and will expect to have this discussion. Do not be shy. It is also important to remember that this is not age related and is a subject which you should expect your doctor to mention.

Q *How long after my treatment will you be able to tell if my cancer is cured?*

A There is no effective evidence of cure. What we can say, however, is that the PSA levels taken after radical surgery would be a very good indication as to the degree of prostate activity left. After radical prostatectomy, the PSA level should be virtually unreadable, i.e. less than 0.1 ng/ml. With radiotherapy, the PSA levels tend to be a bit higher, but it is now accepted at less than 1 ng/ml, or preferably less than 0.5 ng/ml. This is tantamount to a cure. However, PSA levels can come back and if this happens, it is at this stage that hormone therapy might be used.

Q *Are there any new treatments that will become available soon?*

A In the last few years very many new treatments have been appearing in clnical trials and it is likely that at least some of them will find their way into the clinic. Among them is the drug abiraterone acetate, which at the time of writing is still in clinical trials, and it is important that these trials are completed before such drugs are routinely used.

Glossary

Active monitoring The process of observing the patient, giving regular PSA tests, but not actively treating the patient until his symptoms become apparent and require treatment. This form of treatment is valid for many men, who never require radical treatment because they have very slow-growing tumours.

Adenocarcinoma Cancer that appears in glandular tissue such as the prostate.

Adjuvant therapy Treatment given in addition to the primary therapy.

Adrenal androgen A male hormone produced by the adrenal glands; adrenal androgens account for about 5 per cent of the body's androgens.

Advanced prostate cancer Describes the condition where the initial cancer has escaped from the prostate gland to other tissues such as bones and internal organs.

Androgen Male hormone such as testosterone.

Androgen blockade Use of drugs to interrupt the activity of male hormones.

Anti-androgen A drug (usually tablet form) which competes with testosterone and prevents it from functioning.

Benign Describes a tumour that does not invade and destroy the surrounding tissue or migrate to other sites in the body (compare with malignant) and therefore is not cancerous.

Benign prostatic hyperplasia (BPH) A non-malignant enlargement of the prostate which can occur with age.

Biopsy A sample of tissue taken from part of the body (i.e. the prostate gland) which is then analysed under a microscope. A biopsy is normally taken using a small hollow needle.

Bladder neck Thickened muscle where the bladder joins the urethra. On a signal from the brain, this muscle can either tighten or relax to control flow of urine from the bladder to the urethra.

Bladder neck contracture A complication of surgery that causes scarring of the tissue and possible urinary problems. Could require additional surgery to correct.

Bone scan A small harmless amount of radioactive chemical is injected into the body and is taken up by the bones. An image can then be created with cancerous tissue showing up as black spots ('hotspots') on the X-ray film. However, not all hotspots are caused by cancer and you may find some old breaks or previous injuries showing up.

Brachytherapy The implantation of radioactive seeds into the prostate gland. These seeds remain in the prostate and give a continuous low dose of radiation to the cancerous cells. A variation on this is to implant radioactive needles temporarily into the prostate.

Cancer The abnormal and uncontrolled division of cells which may go on to invade and destroy surrounding tissues (see Malignant).

Castration The removal of male hormones either by surgical removal of the testicles or with drugs that inhibit hormone production.

Catheter A tube inserted into a narrow opening or orifice (i.e. in the penis) which allows the release of fluids such as urine.

Chemotherapy The treatment or prevention of disease by the use of chemicals. This term is often used to describe anti-cancer drugs which operate by killing rapidly dividing cells.

Cryotherapy The use of freezing liquids to destroy the prostate gland and eliminate the cancer within it.

CT scan (also CAT; computed axial tomography) A cross-sectional X-ray used in diagnosis and radiation treatment planning.

Cystitis Infection and inflammation of the bladder, which is a possible short-lived side effect of radiation therapy. Causes painful urination.

DES Diethylstilboestrol, a synthetic oestrogen, used in the treatment of prostate cancer.

Differentiated The resemblance of cancer cells to normal cells. Well-differentiated tumour cells closely resemble normal cells and therefore are believed to be less aggressive.

Digital rectal examination (DRE) A simple examination carried out by a doctor or nurse where a gloved finger is placed into the patient's back passage where the prostate gland can be felt for abnormalities.

Dysplasia Abnormal growth of cells.

Dysuria Burning sensation when urinating.

External beam radiotherapy (EBRT) The use of high-energy X-ray beams to target and destroy the cells within the prostate gland and surrounding area.

Flutamide (Eulexin) An anti-androgen used in hormonal treatment.

Frequency The constant need to pass urine, especially at night.

Frozen section A small piece of a larger piece of tissue taken out during a biopsy that is flash frozen for instant analysis by a pathologist using a microscope to determine whether cancer is present.

FSH Follicle-stimulating hormone produced by the pituitary gland to activate sperm-forming tubules in the testicles.

Genes (genetics) All the body's genetic material is in the form of DNA. Lengths of DNA which have a common function, and which code for a particular protein are called genes. When genes become mutated, the resulting proteins are also mutated and may lose their function.

Gene therapy The use of genetic material to prevent or treat disease. This can include introducing genes into cells which cause the destruction of the cell, or introducing genes which activate other cells to kill the cancer.

Gland An organ or group of cells which is specialized for the production of fluids such as semen.

Gleason grade When a biopsy of the prostate is analysed under a microscope, the cells which make up the gland can be examined as to whether they are cancerous based on their size, shape, and structure. A grade can be assigned to the cells (ranging from 1 to 5) which represents how aggressive the cancer may be (see Table 2.1).

Gleason score Two Gleason grades are added together from the two representative parts of the biopsy to give a score, i.e. 2 + 4 = 6 (score out of a possible 10).

Goserelin (Zoladex) A synthetic LHRH agonist/antagonist used in hormonal treatment.

Gray (Gy) A unit of measure for radiation treatment.

Haematuria Blood in the urine

Haemospermia Blood in the sperm.

Hesitancy The need to hesitate before passing urine even when the bladder is full.

HIFU High-frequency ultrasound.

Hormone refractory stage A state where prostate cancer cells no longer require testosterone to grow and therefore grow in its absence. Hormone therapy is no longer effective at this point.

Hormone therapy This can be surgical (where the testicles are removed) or medical (where drugs are given). Both procedures lower the ability of testosterone to feed the cancer.

Hormones Substances which are produced in one part of the body and are carried by the blood to another part where they modify the function or structure of other tissues.

Hot flushes These are flushing and a feeling of temperature change associated with facial flushing.

Hyperplasia Abnormal growth of cells caused by rapid cell multiplication.

Impotence The inability to achieve an erection firm enough for intercourse to take place.

Incontinence Urinary incontinence is the uncontrolled release of urine from the bladder. This usually involves the constant dribbling of urine and sometimes requires that an incontinence pad or sheath be worn in the underwear.

LHRH agonist A drug (usually injected into the abdomen) which causes a reduction in testosterone production.

Libido Sexual drive or sexual desire. This can be affected by treatments which alter testosterone function such as medical hormone therapy or orchidectomy.

Localized prostate cancer A condition where the cancerous tissue is contained within the prostate gland (compare with advanced prostate cancer).

Luteinizing hormone (LH) This hormone is secreted by the pituitary gland. It stimulates secretion of androgen by the testicles.

Luteinizing hormone-releasing hormone (LHRH) This hormone is secreted by the brain to stimulate the secretion of LH by the pituitary gland.

Lymph nodes Small bean-shaped organs located along the lymphatic system. Nodes filter bacteria or cancer cells that may travel through the lymphatic system. Also called lymph glands.

Lymphatic system The tissues and organs, including the bone marrow, spleen, thymus, and lymph nodes, that produce and store cells that fight infection and disease.

MAB (maximal androgen blockade) Hormonal therapy using drugs to block the production and activity of male hormones completely.

Malignant Describes a tumour which has the ability to destroy tissue or spread to distant sites in the body (compare with benign).

Metastases Secondary tumours that have migrated from the prostate gland and become established in other sites in the body.

Nocturia The need to get up frequently at night to urinate.

Oncologist A doctor who specializes in the treatment of cancer.

Orchidectomy An operation in which both testicles, or part of both testicles, are removed in order to prevent production of testosterone.

Palliative Treatment that relieves symptoms such as pain but does not cure.

PIN (prostatic intra-epithelial neoplasia) Believed by some pathologists to be a pre-malignant lesion if it is high grade.

Priapism The presence of an erection persisting for more than 4 hours. Medical attention should be sought if this occurs.

Proctitis Irritation and pain in the rectum and anus, causing diarrhoea and bleeding, a potential side effect of radiation therapy.

Prostate gland A gland that is located beneath the bladder and produces secretions which nourish and protect sperm when ejaculated.

Prostatitis Inflammation of the prostate gland which may be caused by bacterial infection and may respond to antibiotics.

Proteins The building blocks of life. Proteins are made up of amino acids which are pieced together using genes as a template. Proteins form the structural material that makes up the tissues, organs, and muscles as well as forming hormones and other regulatory molecules.

PSA (prostate–specific antigen) A protein found in men which is exclusively produced by the prostate gland. This protein leaks out into the blood where it can be measured.

PSA tests A measurement of PSA in the blood. This level rises when there is a problem with the prostate gland but the test does not differentiate between cancer and other non-malignant conditions.

Radical prostatectomy The complete removal of the prostate gland (compare with TURP).

Radiotherapist A doctor who specializes in radiotherapy in the treatment of disease.

Radiotherapy The use of radiation in the treatment of disease. This radiation can be applied from outside the body (see External beam radiotherapy) or from within the body (see Brachytherapy).

Seminal vesicles Two glands, like small bunches of grapes, at the top of the prostate and behind the bladder which produce the sticky substance in semen.

Staging The process carried out to detect whether a cancer is confined or has spread.

Surgeon A doctor who specializes in carrying out operations. This will usually be a urologist who deals with prostate surgery.

Testosterone A male hormone, which is produced mainly by the testicles and is often responsible for feeding prostate cancer and making it grow.

TRUS (transrectal ultrasound scan) The use of an ultrasound probe (similar to that used in the imaging of unborn babies) which is placed inside the back passage and provides an image of the prostate gland. Often used to guide the needle used for biopsy.

Tumour An abnormal growth of tissue which may be benign or malignant.

TURP (transurethral resection of the prostate) The removal of part of the prostate gland from within the penis. The surgical tool, a resectoscope, is placed inside the penis, down the urethra, where the prostate gland is shaved away from the inside.

Urethra The tube which carries urine from the bladder to the opening of the penis. This tube is surrounded by the prostate gland just below the bladder.

Urologist A doctor who specializes in the treatment of urinary tract diseases such as those affecting the bladder, the prostate, and the tubes which carry urine from the kidneys to the bladder.

Vas deferens Tube through which sperm travels from each testicle to the centre of the prostate in the urethra.

Sources of information

Useful books

Baggish, J. (1995). *Making the Prostate Therapy Decision* (American). Lowell House, Los Angeles, CA (ISBN 1–5656520–7X).

Haig, S. (ed.) (1995). *Understanding Cancer of the Prostate*. London: British Association of Cancer United Patients (CancerBACUP) (ISBN 1–870403–71–1). Available free from BACUP, Tel: (0)20 7696 9003.

Kirk, D. (1995). *Understanding Prostate Disorders*. London: British Medical Association (ISBN 1–898205–14–0).

Korda, M. (1997). *Man to Man* (American). Boston: Little Brown (ISBN 0–316–88297–6).

Loo, M.H. and Betancourt, M. (1998). *The Prostate Cancer Sourcebook*. John Wiley, Chichester (ISBN 0–471–15927–1).

Meyer, S. and Nash, S. (1994). *Prostate Cancer: Making Survival Decisions* (American). University of Chicago Press (ISBN 0–226–56857–1).

Newton, A.C. (1996). *Livin g with Prostate Cancer*. McClelland & Stewart, Toronto (ISBN 0–7710–6779–8).

Phillips, R.H. (1994) *Coping with Prostate Cancer*. Avery, New York (ISBN 0–89529–564–4).

Smith, J. and Gillatt, D. (1996). *Prostate Problems*. Hodder & Stoughton, London (ISBN 0–340–67907–7).

Useful addresses

The Prostate Cancer Charity

First Floor, Cambridge House

100 Cambridge Grove

Hammersmith

London W6 0LE

Tel: 020 8222 7622 (general enquiries and donations)

Fax: 020 8222 7639

Helpline: 0845 300 8383

E-mail: info@prostate-cancer.org.uk

Website: www.prostate-cancer.org.uk

CancerBACUP (British Association of Cancer United Patients)

3 Bath Place

Rivington Street

London EC2A 3JR

Tel: 020 7696 9003

Fax: 020 7696 9002

Helpline: 020 7613 2121 (within London)

Freephone: 0800 18 11 99 (outside London)

Website: www.bacup.org.uk

Cancerlink

11–21 Northdown Street

London N1 9BN

Tel: 020 7833 2818 (Administration)

Fax: 020 7833 4963

Helpline: 0808 808 0000

Website: cancerlink@cancerlink.org.uk

The Impotence Association

PO Box 10296

London SW17 9WH

Helpline: 020 8767 7791

Website: www.impotence.org.uk

The Continence Foundation

307 Hatton Square

16 Baldwins Gardens

London EC1N 7RJ

Tel: 020 7404 6875

Fax: 020 7474 6876

Helpline: 020 7831 9831

Website: www.vois.org.uk/cf

Cancer Research UK

PO Box 123

Lincoln's Inn Fields

London WC2A 3PX

Tel: 020 7242 0200

Fax: 020 7269 3101

Website: www.icnet.uk

Macmillan Cancer Relief

Anchor House

15–19 Britten Street

London SW3 3TZ

Tel: 020 7351 7811

Fax: 020 7376 8098

Helpline: 0845 601 6161

Website: www.macmillan.org.uk

The Prostate Health Council

American Federation of Urologic Disease (AFUD)

300 West Pratt Street, Suite 401

Baltimore, MD 21201

USA

Information: 1–800–242–2383

Support Group Network: 1–800–7866

Patient information

Information booklets by CancerBACUP

Coping at Home
Coping with Hair Loss
Facing the Challenge of Advanced Cancer
Feeling Better
Controlling Pain and other Symptoms of Cancer
Understanding Chemotherapy
Understanding Cancer of the Prostate
Understanding Clinical Trials
Understanding Radiotherapy

Other patient publications

The Cancer Guide. Macmillan Cancer Relief, 15–19 Britten Street, London SW3 3TZ.
Bereavement. Help the Aged, St James Walk, Clerkenwell Green, London EC1R 0BE.

Useful websites

American Cancer Society: http://www.cancer.org

American Urological Association: http://www.auanet.org

Bacup: http://www.cancerbacup.org.uk

Cancer Research Campaign: http://www.crc.org.uk

CaP CURE: http://www.capcure.org

Guide to Internet resources for cancer: http://www.ncl.ac.uk/childhealth/guides/clinks1.html

National Cancer Institute, USA: http://www.nci.nih.gov

SEER Cancer Statistics: http://www.seer.ims.nci.nih.gov

SIECUS: http://www.siecus.org

Us Too! International: http://www.ustoo.com

Index